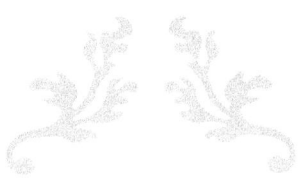

"GOLDEN EGGS" FOR EMPTY NESTERS

Instead of downsizing, turn your home into a "Golden Egg" financially and spiritually, with very little financial investment!

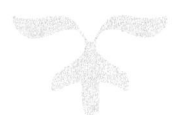

BY
RICK LUNDBERG

"Golden Eggs" for Empty Nesters

Work from home, Using your home!

TABLE OF CONTENTS

Chapter One – THE GOLDEN EGGS
Lottie

Chapter Two - GOALS
Ruthie

Chapter Three - REQUIREMENTS
M

Chapter Four - INVESTMENT
Oesa

Chapter Five – GETTING STARTED
Monica

Chapter Six - CHOOSING A BUSINESS ENTITY
Jim & Gloria

Chapter Seven - REGISTERING YOUR BUSINESS NAME

    Shaley

Chapter Eight - COMPENSATION

    Dad

Chapter Nine – TIME

    Angie

Chapter Ten - BANKING

    Ed

Chapter Eleven - INSURANCE

    Joe

Chapter Twelve - CHOOSING THE LEVEL OF CARE

    Paul

Chapter Thirteen - MARKETING

    Frank

Chapter Fourteen – RESPITE

    Tom

Chapter Fifteen - LONG TERM / SHORT TERM

    A few short-term caregivers

Chapter Sixteen – RESIDENTS

Xavien

Chapter Seventeen – FAMILY

Lili

Chapter Eighteen - CAREGIVERS

Analiza, Isabelle, & Suzanne

Chapter Nineteen – MINISTRY OPPORTUNITIES

Tami

Chapter Twenty - TAXES

Ron

Chapter Twenty-One – WHEN YOU ARE FULL TO CAPACITY

Mickey, David, Elliot, John, John & Pat

Chapter Twenty-Two – EXIT PLAN

Pets

Chapter Twenty-Three – REFERENCES

Summary

Your home is one of the largest investments you have made.

Why trade it in for a smaller model which will have a smaller return on your investment.

SCRIPTURE

James 1:27 NLT

Pure and genuine religion in the sight of God the Father means caring for orphans and widows in their distress and refusing to let the world corrupt you.

James 1:27 NIV

Religion that God our Father accepts as pure and faultless is this: to look after orphans and widows in their distress and keep oneself from being polluted by the world.

YOU MUST LOVE PEOPLE AND HAVE A HEART FOR THE ELDERLY OR THE MENTALLY CHALLENGED TO BE SUCCESSFUL IN THIS BUSINESS.

We chose to care for our residents using an UNLICENSED Residential Eldercare Home. Licensing requirements were extensive and not economically feasible for us. An unlicensed home in Texas can easily have a NET Income of $7,000 per month or more for 3 residents. A licensed home in Texas would need to have 15 residents, just to BREAK EVEN!

This book is about turning your home into an UNLICENSED Residential Eldercare Home.

DEDICATION

This book is dedicated

to

My Wife Marilyn

Who prayed for this answer to our financial future

and to

All those who chose to spend their last days and years with us, and their families who entrusted us with their care

CHAPTER ONE

THE GOLDEN EGGS

Your "Empty Nest" can be filled with several "Golden Eggs". All are extremely important, satisfying and rewarding.

How would you like to earn an extra $9,000, or more, per month, working from your home? Could you use an extra $108,000, or more, per year, for as many years as you would like in the future? Would that help you in your retirement? Would it help you get out of debt and stay out of debt? Would you be able to help out your children and grandchildren financially, whether they needed it or not? Would you like to travel wherever you wanted, and whenever you wanted?

Just imagine that within ten or fifteen years, you could be completely debt free, and possibly have over a million dollars in savings. **That is a Golden Egg!**

Other **Golden Eggs** are revealed throughout this book.

A little about us, and why we do what we do.

When my wife, Marilyn, and I lived in Minnesota we were self-employed entrepreneurs. We were also altar ministers in our church.

I had spent 8 years working as a draftsman and project manager for a nationally honored consulting engineering firm in Minneapolis. I left that firm to become an independent contractor working on specific projects for several firms, including the firm I had just left. I did that part time for the next 12 years.

I had also just opened up a small engraving and jewelry store in a new strip mall near my home. I had been developing that business part time for a few years. After a couple of years in the store, I was finally bringing in more money than it was costing me to be open, as I had been building inventory the entire time. The hours were horrendous and my partner was my ex-wife, so I sold that business.

Then Marilyn and I started a property management and maintenance business, providing services to commercial property owners, including mowing and weed control in the summer, and snow removal in the winter. Many of the properties were vacant properties where either a business had closed, or was waiting to be developed, and usually in urban areas where local ordinances required properties to be maintained. We started with a few properties in the Minneapolis and St Paul area, which the two of us were able to take of ourselves.

Marilyn was able to leave her full-time job and take care of the office part of our business after a couple of years.

Within 3 years, we had 44 crews maintaining properties in 14 states in the Midwest.

As things evolved we began a residential side to our business under another name, after a drought in the region had destroyed many lawns. We bought another truck, some equipment, and began restoring lawns by reseeding them. We then offered fertilizing, weed control, and mowing packages, installing sprinkler systems, and even doing some landscaping. We grew to a client list of around 50 homes and other businesses. By then our sons and some of their friends could help out.

Again, Marilyn and I had some free time on our hands. Sams' Clubs started taking orders from customers who could fax in a list, and it would be ready for them to pick up a few hours later. I approached them, and offered my services to their customers in the Twin City area who would pay me a fee for delivering those orders to them. I bought a delivery truck with an electric lift on the back and went to work. That business I did by myself. Physically it was demanding because people would order large appliances or furniture, and businesses would order pallets of copy paper or other supplies, and everyone wanted their things delivered to their final resting place. Financially it was OK, but nothing to shout about.

During that time, we had opened our large home to do adult foster care for young adults with mental disabilities. We had 2 young men, Dan and John who lived with us for a few years. They both had severe anxiety, compulsive behavior, paranoia and general social behavior problems. We had remodeled the lower part of our home, creating a kitchen, a full bath, a living room, and 2 bedrooms. Dan and John could fix their own meals and could care for themselves with supervision from us. The county paid us for their care. It wasn't a lot, but it paid for our utilities, property taxes, insurance, and what we spent on them.

About that time, Marilyn's mother passed away and her father needed to live with us. The county found new homes for Dan and John. A few months later Marilyn found a townhouse nearby for her father to move into.

We now had some extra time on our hands in the evenings, and began doing street ministry in the drug zone of Minneapolis. We volunteered with a couple of homeless shelters, and one rehab center in the area, a few nights per week. The homeless broke our hearts. Every story was different, but the results were about the same. They suffered from addictions, mental illness, or just plain bad luck. Many lives were affected and several changed, including our own lives over the course of 3 or 4 years.

Marilyn's father passed away during the summer of 1997.

We decided to take an extended vacation in January of 1998 to Texas. There was no snow in San Antonio, so we stayed. We bought a lot and contracted for a house to be built. We closed on the house in July and moved down in November after selling our businesses and our primary home in Minnesota. We still had a home on a lake about 60 miles north of Minneapolis, and a park model RV in a resort community near the Wisconsin border. We intended to use those places in the summer months for fishing, golfing, spending time with our kids, grandchildren, and feeding mosquitoes.

After a few months in Texas we became bored. Doing some ministry at our new church, and a couple of short term mission trips per year didn't keep us busy enough. So, we decided to start up a real estate business. We hired a broker, built a website, and Marilyn and I began buying houses to fix up and sell, or rent out. I eventually got my real estate license, and then a broker's license in Texas. Then I got my real estate license in Minnesota and California, while Marilyn got hers in Texas.

That kept us busy until the real estate bubble burst in 2007. We had just bought and moved into a newly built home in a gated community. The house was a lot larger and nicer than we really needed, but it was a great deal and seemed right at the time.

Marilyn turned to the Lord in prayer as to what we should do. He answered with the scriptures listed at the beginning of this book!

Now let's talk about you!

When many couples become empty nesters they first proclaim their new-found independence, and then begin a grieving period, followed by loneliness, then a desire to downsize their living requirements to save both housework, yard work, and money.

These days both husband and wife have been working to provide for their family. Most are employees working for someone else in an hourly or a salaried position. Some are self-employed owners of a small business.

At this time in their life, they have the opportunity to plan for their own future. Empty nesters may be looking forward to someday retiring, or at least cutting back their workload. But, in many cases have not been able to set aside enough money to do so in the near future.

Every generation is getting older. Many elderly persons are still quite able to care for themselves without assistance. Many others are taking care of their spouses whose health is deteriorating, either mentally, physically, or both. As they retire, they are eligible for benefits, Social Security, pensions, disability compensation, or perhaps they were able to set aside funds for Long Term Care.

When those persons can no longer safely care for themselves, the families usually step in and **if possible**, take on that responsibility. If they are unable, or unwilling to take on that 24 hours per day task, they start looking for a place that can.

Large assisted living facilities are generally the first place they look, especially if the person qualifies for an insurance plan to help with cost, or if the family is not aware of other options. The family may have already used meals on wheels, or had someone come in to their home for a few hours a week to help with chores, or prepare a few meals.

Our experience with large facilities has led us to believe that residents become room or bed numbers, and sometimes wear ankle bracelets with GPS tags so staff can find them more easily. The ratio for residents to caregivers is also quite high.

A **Residential Eldercare** home is a place where residents can be treated like family, in a comfortable, non-sterile environment. They get a private room, and sometimes a private bath. They may have some of their own bedroom furniture, a few of their favorite pictures on the wall, and a sense of security with familiar objects and surroundings.

Residential Eldercare homes provide the owners with both something to do, and additional income, all at home. **Golden Egg!**

LOTTIE

Lottie was one of our first residents. She lived alone after her husband past away for several years. Her son lived in Atlanta, and could not visit often. He called us to see if we could care for his mother, as her neighbors were concerned for her safety. She was 92 years old, and was a retired school teacher, who taught art. Her mind was clear, but her body was failing. We met with her and showed her our home, and explained to her what we could do to make her life easier.

We moved her in, and encouraged her to stay as active as she could. She kept busy crocheting small items, and gave them to her friend, who was a chaplain in a pediatric cancer hospital. Her friend and her friend's husband would visit every couple of months, and bring back to the hospital, the boxes of items that Lottie had made, and boxes of toys that we collected from Kid's Meals at the local fast food chains. My wife and I were, and still are, real estate professionals, so we ate fast food a lot back then.

Whenever she needed outside medical attention for something, she would always tell us "Don't let them keep me!" We promised we wouldn't and we kept that promise. She always called my wife "Dearie" and referred to me as "The Man". Marilyn was doing the majority of caregiving at that point. I was a full-time real estate broker, and spent most of my time working out of the house. When we went to church, she always enjoyed going with us.

After living with us past her 96th birthday, she took a turn for the worse. Hospice nurses came to our home every day, sometimes several times a day, for several weeks, to help us care for her, and give her medications to comfort her.

Toward the end, the only food she wanted to eat was vanilla ice cream. Which worked out well, as we could crush up her pills, and mix them into the ice cream. One afternoon, after I had fed her some ice cream, she simply stated she wanted to take a nap, and passed away peacefully in her sleep.

Her son was very grateful for the care we had provided. Marilyn sent her very personal things to him, and at his suggestion, donated the rest to the Salvation Army.

CHAPTER TWO

GOALS

Financial -   Many empty nesters spend more money on their kids, AFTER they leave home. Between college and periods of unemployment and underemployment, they might still need some additional help.

How much additional income will you require for your immediate, short term, and your retirement needs?

Could you use a **"Golden Egg"** to pay off your mortgage and other debt?

Here is one scenario: Tom and Sue just had Tom Junior leave home. Junior just graduated from college, and has accepted an entry level position in his field, in a different community. For a while he needed some financial help until he got promoted. Tom and Sue decided that a little extra money might come in handy. The assisted living facility near Tom and Sue charges $4,000 per month as a base level fee. Charges go up as the level of required care goes up.

Tom and Sue have a 4-bedroom home, and determined that if they provided a place for 2 residents at $3,000 per month, they would have $6,000 additional monthly income. They will now have one additional room for a live-in caregiver (Debby). If they provide Debby with free room and board (which has a lot of value) and have her work 2 days and 2 nights per week, they will have no extra out of pocket expenses, for Debby, other than food.

So now the expenses will be food, a little extra utility expenses, and insurance. Even if Debby works some additional days per month at $60 per day, the expenses are around $1,500 per month. That leaves an additional net income of $4,500 per month. Of course, that is taxable income to them through their LLC. However, they now use 60% of their home for business purposes, and they are able to deduct 60% of ALL their expenses for their home, on their income tax return. They are having their accountant/tax preparer handle that. It will be 15 years until they retire, and they intend to do this until then.

They could also choose to rent out the 60% of their home to the LLC and show the income and deductions on their personal IRS Form 1040 tax return.

See the chapter on Taxes for more information.

If you could use an extra $810,000 toward helping your kids and your retirement, you might consider this. This does not account for inflation, or additional residents. **Golden Egg!**

Careful though! Most states require a license to operate a Residential Eldercare Home, or an Assisted Living facility, after you reach a certain number of residents. Check with your own states regulations. See the list at the end of this book for information as of the date of publishing.

RUTHIE

Ruthie came to live with us shortly after Lottie moved in. Her daughter lived a few miles away, so our large home was convenient. Ruthie was physically in fairly good shape, and ambulatory, considering she was an 80-something. However, her dementia was at a point where she could not live alone, and her family could not care for her 24/7.

Ruthie and Lottie quickly became friends. Ruthie's dementia was quite sweet, to match her personality. Every meal was a brand-new experience. Every animal was a "Kitty"; including several deer in the neighborhood, that would come into our back yard for some dried corn, which we would spread out in the evening, as we sat on the deck off the kitchen.

After a couple of years Ruthie's needs, and NEW aggressive behaviors required additional medications and care, according to her doctor, who we agreed with. However, her daughter didn't think that treatment plan was necessary for her mom. Safety concerns for ourselves, our caregivers, and other residents, made it necessary for us to notify Ruthie's family that we could no longer take care of her in our home.

Her daughter moved her into a large facility for seniors. However, we learned later, that it was under the conditions that the Doctors and Nurses would be in charge of her care. Ruthie got what SHE needed, but her quality of life was diminished in that institutional environment.

CHAPTER THREE

REQUIREMENTS

The main requirement is your personal desire to help and care for elderly men, or women, who desperately need help. Patience and tolerance are a big help also. It wouldn't hurt if at least one of you has had some caregiving experience in the past. My wife was a CNA for three years in a hospital.

The next requirement is a home you can share, 24/7, with those who need help.

The home needs to be clean, well maintained, and able to access easily by the elderly. The entrance should be level, or with very few steps, and perhaps a ramp if necessary.

Unlicensed Residential Eldercare Home

vs

Licensed Assisted Living or Nursing Homes

The decision for us to choose **NOT to be licensed was EASY** no matter how many or how few residents we can care for. See the chapter on References for your states requirements.

Here in Texas we are allowed to care for up to 3 persons who are not related to us without being licensed.

SOME of the requirements for complying with licensing may include the following:

- Your home must have a fire suppression or sprinkler system throughout your home.
- You must have a licensed nursing professional on duty 24/7/365.
- You must have a doctor on call if needed.
- You must have a dietician overseeing all menus and meal preparation activities.
- Your entire facility must be ADA compliant.
- You must accept insurance or government payments as part or all of your compensation.
- You must obtain all local permits and have inspections on a regular basis.
- You must maintain complete records and files on all employees and residents.

I did the math!!!! I would need to have 15 residents, JUST TO BREAK EVEN!

I mentioned that fact to one of my realtor/investors. He bought a larger motel and is doing quite well now, but, it took a while to get over the curve.

A desirable floor plan would be open, and well-lit with natural light. Hallways should be wide enough to accommodate 2 people side by side, or a wheel chair. It should also have easy access to a private, or common bathroom with roll-in, or walk-in shower. The dining area needs to be large enough for everyone to sit around the table, and a living area where residents and caregivers can sit, talk, read, or watch TV.

Make sure you have a place outdoors, that is fairly secure, for your residents to enjoy. A relatively level, hard surface such as a deck or patio, with shade and places to sit and rest will attract a resident. Maybe a bird feeder and some hanging baskets for flowers would be nice too. You could also plant some tomatoes or other fruits and vegetables in containers.

As a general rule, a swimming pool is not a good idea, unless it is completely secured from unsupervised use.

Typically, our residents tend to be more comfortable with a little warmer environment, so our heat is set at 73, and our A/C is set at 77. So, we just set the thermostat to AUTO, and leave it there.

Lastly, the vehicle you use to transport the residents to appointments, outings, or church needs to be easily accessible, well maintained and insured, with responsible drivers operating the vehicle.

M

M was short for Marilyn, but this Marilyn was a younger woman who came to help us care for our residents. As 24/7/365 caregiving responsibilities had taken a toll on my wife and I.

M moved into one of the bedrooms on the main level of our home, close to the ladies. She was a writer that worked from home, researching, and writing magazine articles for trade magazines. All she needed from us was internet service, board and room, and some cash. She was wonderful with the ladies. She would even take them grocery shopping with her. We furnished the car, and kept it fully insured, and full of gas. She prepared all the meals on her days to work, kept the house clean and orderly, and kept the ladies entertained. She stayed with us for well over a year before moving on. But, she didn't leave until we had found another live-in caregiver.

CHAPTER FOUR
INVESTMENT

The financial investment is relatively small for starting up your own small business. See the chapter for business entities. It can range from a few hundred dollars, to a few thousand dollars, using a professional to help you prepare and file the documents.

Perhaps a few modifications or improvements to your home would be required.

The personal time investment can be little more than when you were raising your own family, or less if you can accommodate room for a live-in caregiver (see chapter on caregivers) to assist you with the resident's care.

Chances are, you will be involved on a daily basis, until you are comfortable with your caregiver's ability to handle most of the duties and situations that may arise.

If this will be a short-term adventure for you, keep your immediate investment as small as possible. You can always change your mind and go long-term later, when you see how easy this business can be.

Few businesses offer more return for your investment (ROI) than this one! **Golden Egg!**

OESA

Oesa was placed into our home through a referral agency. Her niece had been caring for her prior to that. Oesa was diagnosed with dementia at the early age of 59, and she was 65 when she arrived at our home. She was originally from West Virginia, the youngest daughter in a large coal mining family. She was a brilliant artist who went to college on a scholarship and earned a degree in Art. But now she just used crayons to create her works.

She was quiet and had a few quirks. Since her niece was very busy, and her closest relatives didn't live nearby, I took her to appointments, picked up meds, and whenever necessary we took her to the hospital. She was very sweet, but had an aggressive side that came out when she became frustrated and confused.

One day after breakfast as she was getting up from her chair, she caught her foot on the leg of the chair, fell and fractured her hip. We played back the video surveillance for that area of the home to confirm what had happened. We took her to the ER. After the doctors treated her, she developed complications. Doctors recommended that she be transferred to a skilled nursing facility for Hospice. Since her relatives wanted to come to town and stay with her these last days, they placed her in a facility that could accommodate them as well.

After a few days, my wife, Marilyn, called her niece to see if we could visit. She said that Oesa had not been responsive to anyone since they placed her there, but we would be welcome to visit. We went there right away. When we arrived, Oesa was lying on her right side, the way she would always lay while sleeping. Marilyn walked over to her right side, took her hand, squeezed it, and said "Hi Oesa, it's Marilyn". Oesa squeezed back. Then I walked over to her left side and said "How are you doing Oesa?" She rolled over, opened her eyes and said, "Where have you been?" I said "I'm sorry Oesa, but I've been working." Oesa said "You're always working." I replied, "I know, I'm sorry". Then she said "I love you". I replied, "I know you do Oesa, we love you too". She rolled back over toward Marilyn. Her niece looked at us at amazement and said, "She hasn't moved or said anything to anyone". Oesa passed away several days later, never responding to anyone again.

Oesa had lived with us for nearly 3 years. She never called me by name, but she called Marilyn, "My Angel".

CHAPTER FIVE
GETTING STARTED

Discuss in detail, and Pray about this commitment with your spouse, and other friends or family members who may come to visit, or stay for a while.

Investigate any licensing requirements there may be for your state, or local government, or any deed restrictions, such as a homeowner or property association.

Write a realistic business plan. Do a 10-year, a 5-year, and a 1-year plan, setting personal and business goals. These plans should be reviewed and updated annually.

Have Quickbooks, or other accounting software to do your bookkeeping. Quickbooks will work with Turbo Tax software, when it is time to do your taxes. With these software programs, you can probably do everything yourself. If not, you can pass these reports on to your tax preparer. Make sure you keep accurate records. Quickbooks also can download your banking information, with a little setup from you. You will have to manually enter in any cash transactions and receipts.

Check out some of the assisted living facilities in your area. Find out what they charge for care if you can. Also, check nursing homes in your area. You will find that fees and other charges will vary greatly, depending on amenities offered at each facility.

The best way to start is with ambulatory, minimal assistance required residents. You provide the home, control their medications, prepare all the meals, and see that they remain safe, and groomed.

Your residents will become family, and should be treated as such. Family members don't always see eye to eye on everything, but they still live together, and need to be in a peaceful and safe environment.

I have often said "Eldercare is a lot like daycare for children, only the diapers are bigger."

The hardest part of this business is dealing with family members and finding really good caregivers.

MONICA

Monica responded to an ad Marilyn ran on Craigslist for a live-in caregiver. She needed to be closer to San Antonio, as she had just made the cut to be a Silver Dancer for the San Antonio Spurs NBA team. They don't pay much, so our position looked very good to her.

She had experience caring for her Grandmother, and did a fine interview with us. Again, Monica was great with our residents. She was conscientious and responsible.

We were able to work around her schedule with the Spurs, since we had additional caregiver help at the same time. That worked out great, because we had season tickets to the Spurs, and needed someone to cover for us on game nights as well.

She and Marilyn became very close. Monica came from a dysfunctional family, and needed a motherly figure, and counselor in her life. When Monica got promoted to choreographer for the Austin Toros (now the Austin Spurs) at the beginning of the next season, she had to move back to Austin. But, before she left, Monica filled our caregiver needs with three of the newest Spurs Silver Dancers.

Monica has called and visited Marilyn several times over the past few years, bringing Marilyn flowers, and on one of her last visits, brought along a young man she was dating to see if we approved of him. Not sure what happened to him.

CHAPTER SIX
CHOOSING A BUSINESS ENTITY

These are the most common types of business entities here in the United States. If you are outside of the United States or one of the US territories, you will have to do that research on your own.

Sole Proprietor:

From: Entrepenuer.com

Definition: *A business that legally has no separate existence from its owner. Income and losses are taxed on the individual's personal income tax return.*

The sole proprietorship is the simplest business form under which one can operate a business. The sole proprietorship is not a legal entity. It simply refers to a person who owns the business and is personally responsible for its debts. A sole proprietorship can operate under the name of its owner or it can do business under a fictitious name, such as Nancy's Nail Salon. The fictitious name is simply a trade name--it does not create a legal entity separate from the sole proprietor owner.

The sole proprietorship is a popular business form due to its simplicity, ease of setup, and nominal cost. A sole proprietor need only register his or her name and secure local licenses, and the sole proprietor is ready for business. A distinct disadvantage, however, is that the owner of a sole proprietorship remains personally liable for all the business's debts. So, if a sole proprietor business runs into financial trouble, creditors can bring lawsuits against the business owner. If such suits are successful, the owner will have to pay the business debts with his or her own money.

The owner of a sole proprietorship typically signs contracts in his or her own name, because the sole proprietorship has no separate identity under the law. The sole proprietor owner will typically have customers write checks in the owner's name, even if the business uses a fictitious name. Sole proprietor owners can, and often do, commingle personal and business property and funds, something that partnerships, LLCs and corporations cannot do. Sole proprietorships often have their bank accounts in the name of the owner. Sole proprietors need not observe formalities such as voting and meetings associated with the more complex business forms. Sole proprietorships can bring lawsuits (and can be sued) using the name of the sole proprietor owner. Many businesses begin as sole proprietorships and graduate to more complex business forms as the business develops.

Because a sole proprietorship is indistinguishable from its owner, sole proprietorship taxation is quite simple. The income earned by a sole proprietorship is income earned by its owner. A sole proprietor reports the sole proprietorship income and/or losses and expenses by filling out and filing a Schedule C, along with the standard Form 1040. Your profits and losses are first recorded on a tax form called Schedule C, which is filed along with your 1040. Then the "bottom-line amount" from Schedule C is transferred to your personal tax return. This aspect is attractive because business losses you suffer may offset income earned from other sources.

As a sole proprietor, you must also file a Schedule SE with Form 1040. You use Schedule SE to calculate how much self-employment tax you owe. You need not pay unemployment tax on yourself, although you must pay unemployment tax on any employees of the business. Of course, you won't enjoy unemployment benefits should the business suffer.

Sole proprietors are personally liable for all debts of a sole proprietorship business. Let's examine this more closely because the potential liability can be alarming. Assume that a sole proprietor borrows money to operate but the business loses its major customer, goes out of business, and is unable to repay the loan. The sole proprietor is liable for the amount of the loan, which can potentially consume all her personal assets.

Imagine an even worse scenario: The sole proprietor (or even one her employees) is involved in a business-related accident in which someone is injured or killed. The resulting negligence case can be brought against the sole proprietor owner and against her personal assets, such as her bank account, her retirement accounts, and even her home.

Consider the preceding paragraphs carefully before selecting a sole proprietorship as your business form. Accidents do happen, and businesses go out of business all the time. Any sole proprietorship that suffers such an unfortunate circumstance is likely to quickly become a nightmare for its owner.

If a sole proprietor is wronged by another party, he can bring a lawsuit in his own name. Conversely, if a corporation or LLC is wronged by another party, the entity must bring its claim under the name of the company.

The advantages of a sole proprietorship include:

- Owners can establish a sole proprietorship instantly, easily and inexpensively.
- Sole proprietorships carry little, if any, ongoing formalities.
- A sole proprietor need not pay unemployment tax on himself or herself (although he or she must pay unemployment tax on employees).
- Owners may freely mix business or personal assets.

The disadvantages of a sole proprietorship include:

- Owners are subject to unlimited personal liability for the debts, losses and liabilities of the business.
- Owners cannot raise capital by selling an interest in the business.
- Sole proprietorships rarely survive the death or incapacity of their owners and so do not retain value.

One of the great features of a sole proprietorship is the simplicity of formation. Little more than buying and selling goods or services is needed. In fact, no formal filing or event is required to form a sole proprietorship; it is a status that arises automatically from one's business activity.

Limited Liability Company or LLC

From: Entrepeneur.com

Definition: *A form of business organization with the liability-shield advantages of a corporation and the flexibility and tax pass-through advantages of a partnership.*

Many states allow a business form called the limited liability company (LLC). The LLC arose from business owners' desire to adopt a business structure permitting them to operate like a traditional partnership. Their goal was to distribute income to the partners (who reported it on their individual income tax returns) but also to protect themselves from personal liability for the business's debts, as with the corporate business form. In general, unless the business owner establishes a separate corporation, the owner and partners (if any) assume complete liability for all debts of the business. Under the LLC rules, however, an individual isn't responsible for the firm's debt, provided he or she didn't secure them personally, as with a second mortgage, a personal credit card or by putting personal assets on the line.

The LLC offers a number of advantages over subchapter S corporations. For example, while S corporations can issue only one class of the company stock, LLCs can offer several different classes with different rights. In addition, S corporations are limited to a maximum of 75 individual shareholders (who must be U.S. residents), whereas an unlimited number of individuals, corporations, and partnerships may participate in an LLC.

The LLC also carries significant tax advantages over the limited partnership. For instance, unless the partner in a limited partnership assumes an active role, his or her losses are considered passive losses and cannot be used as tax deductions to offset active income. But if the partner takes an active role in the firm's management, he or she becomes liable for the firm's debt. It's a catch-22 situation. The owners of an LLC, on the other hand, do not assume liability for the business' debt, and any losses the LLC incurs can be used as tax deductions against active income.

However, in exchange for these two considerable benefits, the owners of LLCs must meet the "transferability restriction test," which means the ownership interests in the LLC are not transferable without restriction. This restriction makes the LLC structure unworkable for major corporations. For corporations to attract large sums of capital, their corporate stock must be easily transferable in the stock exchanges. However, this restriction isn't as problematic for smaller companies, where stock ownership transfers take place relatively infrequently.

Since the LLC is a relatively new legal form for businesses, federal and state governments are still looking at ways to tighten regulations concerning them. Unfortunately, some investment promoters use LLCs to evade securities laws. That's why it's imperative to consult with your attorney and CPA before deciding which corporate structure makes sense for your business.

Limited Partnership or LP

From: Entrepeneur.com

Definition: *A business organization that allows limited partners to enjoy limited personal liability while general partners have unlimited personal liability.*

A limited partnership is similar to a general partnership except that it has two classes of partners. The general partner(s) have full management and control of the partnership business but also accept full personal responsibility for partnership liabilities. Limited partners have no personal liability beyond their investment in the partnership interest. Limited partners cannot participate in the general management and daily operations of the partnership business without being considered general partners in the eyes of the law.

The general partner can be either an individual or a corporation. One of the more common limited partnership situations involves a silent partner, where one or more limited partners provide financing for the venture and the general partners run the business. A limited partnership in this case protects the assets of silent partners by limiting their exposure and liability and acts as a conduit to pass current operating profits or losses on to them.

Most jurisdictions require limited partnership agreements to be in writing and, for the most part, contain the same provisions as those in a general partnership agreement-with some complex additions. Legal costs of forming a limited partnership can be even higher than for a corporation because in some states they are governed by securities laws.

Another aspect of limited partnerships is that in some businesses, the limited partner (also called the passive investor) may be subject to special tax liabilities that can offset the tax shelter advantages. The IRS tends to look at these facts on a case-by-case basis.

Limited partnerships file an IRS Form 1065 once a year. Individual limited and general partners include their allocable share of partnership income or loss on their individual income tax returns and pay taxes on that share based on their tax bracket. Partners cannot deduct losses greater than their basis in the partnership, which includes their investment plus any funds loaned to the partnership (except for real estate limited partnerships that are governed by special rules).

The 1986 Tax Reform Act limited the amount of losses a limited partner can deduct on a personal tax return. If the partnership is expected to generate tax losses in its early years, your CPA can help determine whether those losses will benefit you.

S Corporation

From: Entrepeneur.com

Definition: *A special form of corporation that allows the protection of limited liability but direct flow-through of profits and losses.*

The S corporation is often more attractive to small-business owners than a standard (or C) corporation. That's because an S corporation has some appealing tax benefits and still provides business owners with the liability protection of a corporation. With an S corporation, income and losses are passed through to shareholders and included on their individual tax returns. As a result, there's just one level of federal tax to pay.

A corporation must meet certain conditions to be eligible for a subchapter S election. First, the corporation must have no more than 75 shareholders. In calculating the 75-shareholder limit, a husband and wife count as one shareholder. Also, only the following entities may be shareholders: individuals, estates, certain trusts, certain partnerships, tax-exempt charitable organizations, and other S corporations (but only if the other S corporation is the sole shareholder).

In addition, owners of S corporations who don't have inventory can use the cash method of accounting, which is simpler than the accrual method. Under this method, income is taxable when received and expenses are deductible when paid.

S corporations do come with some downsides. For example, S corporations are subject to make of the same requirements corporations must follow, and that means higher legal and tax service costs. They also must file articles of incorporation, hold directors and shareholder's meetings, keep corporate minutes, and allow shareholders to vote on major corporate decisions. The legal and accounting costs of setting up an S corporation are also similar to those for a standard corporation. And S corporations can only issue common stock, which can hamper capital-raising efforts.

A corporation must make the subchapter S election no later than two months and 15 days after the first day of the taxable year to elect. Subchapter S election requires the consent of all shareholders.

The states treat S corporations differently. Some states disregard subchapter S status entirely, offering no tax break at all. Other states honor the federal election automatically. Finally, some states require the filing of a state-specific form to complete subchapter S election. Consult an attorney in your state to determine the rules that apply to your business.

An S corporation may revoke its subchapter S status by either failing to meet the conditions of eligibility for S corporations, or by filing with the IRS no later than two months and 15 days after the first day of the taxable year. Once the revocation becomes effective, the business will be taxed as a corporation.

When it comes to choosing the best structure for a business, many entrepreneurs have trouble making a choice between S corporations and LLCs--that's most likely because they possess similarities: They offer their owners limited liability protection and are both pass-through tax entities. Pass-through taxation allows the income or loss generated by the business to be reflected on the personal income tax return of the owners. This special tax status eliminates any possibility of double taxation for S corporations and LLCs.

That's where the similarities end. The ownership of an S corporation is restricted to no more than 75 shareholders, whereas an LLC can have an unlimited number of members (owners). And while an S corporation can't have non-U.S. citizens as shareholders, an LLC can. In addition, S corporations cannot be owned by C corporations, other S corporations, many trusts, LLCs or partnerships. LLCs are not subject to these restrictions.

LLCs are also more flexible in distributing profits than S corporations, wherein the corporation can only have one class of stock and your percentage of ownership determines the percentage of pass-through income. On the other hand, an LLC can have many different classes of interest, and the percentage of pass-through income is not tied to ownership percentage. The pass-through percentage can be set by agreement of the members in the LLC's operating agreement.

S corporations aren't without their advantages, however. One person can form an S corporation, while in a few states at least two people are required to form an LLC. Existence is perpetual for S corporations. Conversely, LLCs typically have limited life spans.

The stock of S corporations is freely transferable, while the interest (ownership) of LLCs is not. This free transferability of interest means the shareholders of S corporations are able to sell their interest without obtaining the approval of the other shareholders. In contrast, member of LLCs would need the approval of the other members in order to sell their interest. Lastly, S corporations may be advantageous in terms of self-employment taxes in comparison to LLCs.

For more information on the rules that apply to a Subchapter S corporation, talk with your CPA.

C Corporation

From: Entrepeneur.com

Definition: *A form of business operation that declares the business as a separate, legal entity guided by a group of officers known as the board of directors.*

A corporate structure is perhaps the most advantageous way to start a business because the corporation exists as a separate entity. In general, a corporation has all the legal rights of an individual, except for the right to vote and certain other limitations. Corporations are given the right to exist by the state that issues their charter. If you incorporate in one state to take advantage of liberal corporate laws but do business in another state, you'll have to file for "qualification" in the state in which you wish to operate the business. There's usually a fee that must be paid to qualify to do business in a state.

You can incorporate your business by filing articles of incorporation with the appropriate agency in your state. Usually, only one corporation can have any given name in each state. After incorporation, stock is issued to the company's shareholders in exchange for the cash or other assets they transfer to it in return for that stock. Once a year, the shareholders elect the board of directors, who meet to discuss and guide corporate affairs anywhere from once a month to once a year.

Each year, the directors elect officers such as a president, secretary and treasurer to conduct the day-to-day affairs of the corporate business. There also may be additional officers such as vice presidents, if the directors so decide. Along with the articles of incorporation, the directors and shareholders usually adopt corporate bylaws that govern the powers and authority of the directors, officers and shareholders.

Even small, private, professional corporations, such as a legal or dental practice, need to adhere to the principles that govern a corporation. For instance, upon incorporation, common stock needs to be distributed to the shareholders and a board of directors elected. If there's only one person forming the corporation, that person is the sole shareholder of stock in the corporation and can elect himself or herself to the board of directors as well as any other individuals that person deems appropriate.

Corporations, if properly formed, capitalized and operated (including appropriate annual meetings of shareholders and directors) limit the liability of their shareholders. Even if the corporation is not successful or is held liable for damages in a lawsuit, the most a shareholder can lose is his or her investment in the stock. The shareholder's personal assets are not on the line for corporate liabilities.

Corporations file Form 1120 with the IRS and pay their own taxes. Salaries paid to shareholders who are employees of the corporation are deductible. But dividends paid to shareholders aren't deductible and therefore don't reduce the corporation's tax liability. A corporation must end its tax year on December 31 if it derives its income primarily from personal services (such as dental care, legal counseling, business consulting and so on) provided by its shareholders.

If the corporation is small, the shareholders should prepare and sign a shareholders buy-sell agreement. This contract provides that if a shareholder dies or wants to sell his or her stock, it must first be offered to the surviving shareholders. It also may provide for a method to determine the fair price that should be paid for those shares. Such agreements are usually funded with life insurance to purchase the stock of deceased shareholders.

If a corporation is large and sells its shares to many individuals, it may have to register with the Securities and Exchange Commission (SEC) or state regulatory bodies. More common is the corporation with only a few shareholders, which can issue its shares without any such registration under private offering exemptions. For a small corporation, responsibilities of the shareholders can be defined in the corporate minutes, and a shareholder who wants to leave can be accommodated without many legal hassles. Also, until your small corporation has operated successfully for many years, you will most likely still have to accept personal liability for any loans made by banks or other lenders to your corporation.

While some people feel that a corporation enhances the image of a small business, one disadvantage is the potential double taxation: The corporation must pay taxes on its net income, and shareholders must also pay taxes on any dividends received from the corporation. Business owners often increase their own salaries to reduce or wipe out corporate profits and thereby lower the possibility of having those profits taxed twice-once to the corporation and again to the shareholders upon receipt of dividends from the corporation.

Other legal entities you might want to know about:

Living Trust

From: Duhaime.org

Living Trust Definition: *A trust from persons to take effect during their living years, to benefit others.*

Related Terms: Revocable Trust, Inter Vivos, Testamentary Trust

Distinguished from the more common trust created by will, which only takes effect upon the death of the person creating the trust (known in law as the settlor, donor or *grantor*). In a *living trust*, the transfer of property occurs inter vivos; between persons living; many jurists refer to the *living trust* by the term inter vivos trust.

In 1998, in a case known in the law reports as Limb v Aldridge, Justice Carl Jones of the Court of Civil Appeals of Oklahoma wrote:

"[A] living trust is a trust which takes effect during the life of the settlor, as distinguished from a testamentary trust which is created upon the settlor's death....

" [A] revocable living trust in which the trustor declares himself trustee and also sole beneficiary of the trust income during his life has been widely promoted as a *will substitute* which purports to avoid the time and expense of probate."

In Weber v Langholz, Justice Vogel of the Court of Appeals of California noted:

"[A] revocable living trust with the settlor as trustee has become a common device for people to manage their own assets during lifetime, avoid having to establish a conservatorship in the event of incapacity, and avoid probate upon death....

[T]he settlors of a revocable living trust (have) a reversionary interest in the subject property...."

Since the *living trust* is often used to benefit family members, it is also referred to as a *family trust*. Historically, families would create *living trusts* at the time of marriage of their children for the prospective benefit of their grandchildren. In the Limb case cited above, the trust was described as follows:

"Virgil R. Limb executed a document creating the Limb Revocable Living Trust in April, 1994, designating himself as trustee (and his daughter as alternate trustee). The two named beneficiaries were his children by a former marriage. Father transferred all of his real and personal property to Trust: his checking account, a small insurance policy, some stocks and bonds, and a car."

Probate and estate taxes can often take a huge bite out of a person's assets at the time of death and so to keep as much money within the family as possible, the tool of a *living trust* is used.

Living trusts can be revocable by the settlor or irrevocable, with, typically, beneficial tax treatment reserved only for irrevocable *living trusts*.

Generally speaking, at any one moment in time, tax authorities are a step behind the craftiness of *living trust* makers (i.e. lawyers) but tax treatment of *living trusts* have, for the most part, caught up in substance if not in detail. If it moves and jingles, the tax man will sooner or later, make an appearance.

Tax treatment can take the form of segregating the trust for tax purposes; it has its own tax return and is taxed separately; or the treatment of the trust as an extension and part of the taxable assets of the beneficiary. In terms of personal income tax, the trick is to transfer within the limits without triggering taxation on the amount so-flowing. This may, for example, take the form of a gift transfer deduction or exemption, which is recorded in a separate tax form.

Another example of a living trust would be elder grandfather, let's call him *Rich Grandpa Settlor* who wants to gift his grand-daughter, *Flighty Ms Beneficiary* but wants to control the flow of the asset to her. He sets us a *living trust* and pours $1-million into it, appointing his eldest son *Mr. Mature Trustee* as, well, trustee. It is declared to be irrevocable which means even if Flighty Ms Beneficiary becomes an axe-murderess or drug addict, Rich Grandpa Settlor is out the cash in any event. The trust is set to end when the money has been evenly distributed under the administration of Flighty Ms Beneficiarys' uncle Mr. Mature Trustee, and Mr. Mature Trustee should be called King Trustee, as he has discretion over much of the trust.

Often, but not always, the trust is named after the beneficiary, as in the "Ms Sally Watson Trust".

Trusts are popular with lawyers because they are so flexible. They allow the transfer of assets from a person to a trust in so many different ways and with an almost unlimited variety of conditions and terms. And so all *living trusts* are different and adjusted to the needs of the settlor and his/her beneficiary and, to a lesser degree, to the abilities of the trustee. In some cases, the settlor, for the duration of his life anyway, or the trustee(s), may also be the beneficiaries.

If you really took the time to read about all of these entities, you realize that each of these have many pros and cons to consider.

In my personal case, I chose not to use sole proprietor as a business form for liability concerns. Especially when caring for residents who may be ambulatory, but may accidentally fall and injure themselves or others.

My personal situation is not complex, but my business model is. I use a combination of all of these except the S Corporation, as my wife and I have small businesses in Texas, Nevada, and Minnesota

I personally would recommend using a Limited Liability Company (LLC) for any small business of this nature.

If you or your attorney do not know what a charging order is, find an attorney that does. That one section of your corporate documents, could keep you from being sued for any reason what-so-ever!

From nolo.com:

Charging Orders

All states permit personal creditors of an LLC owner to obtain a charging order against the debtor-owner's membership interest. A charging order is an order issued by a court directing an LLC's manager to pay to the debtor-owner's personal creditor any distributions of income or profits that would otherwise be distributed to the debtor-member.

However, in most states, creditors with a charging order only obtain the owner-debtor's "financial rights" and cannot participate in management of the LLC. Thus, the creditor cannot order the LLC to make a distribution subject to its charging order. Very frequently, creditors who obtain charging orders end up with nothing because they can't order the LLC to make any distributions. As a result, they are not a very effective collection tool for creditors.

Example: The collection agency obtains a charging order from a court ordering the Acme LLC to pay to it any distributions of money or property the LLC would ordinarily make to John until the entire $38,000 judgment is paid. However, if there are no distributions, there will be no payments.

The charging order remedy without any right to order distributions is so weak, many creditors don't even try to use it.

In about half the states, the charging order is the exclusive (only) legal remedy personal creditors of LLC members have.

MY OPINION WHY the CHARGING ORDER PROTECTS YOU SO WELL –

Suppose someone files a suit against your LLC, FOR ANY REASON, and the court sides with them, and awards them $200,000. The general partner in the LLC is only liable for his percentage of the award. Let's say the general partner has 5% of the shares. He is only liable for $10,000. But he can legally choose to not pay it, if he doesn't want to.

However, because the suit was awarded to the plaintiff, and the court has notified the IRS of the award as income to the plaintiff and their legal representatives, the IRS will be looking for that income on their income tax returns as if they had actually gotten the money. And they would be legally required to pay that tax as if they had actually gotten it.

The attorneys know this, and in this scenario, will not want to file the suit, and take a chance on owing the IRS taxes on $60,000 or so, that they never received.

Now that's a **GOLDEN EGG** too. And probably the best protection against ever being sued.

My advice – form another LLC to protect your personal assets, such as bank accounts, real estate, jewelry, fine arts, securities, and anything else of value. You don't have to deed them over, just list them in Schedule A of the LLC documents and record them at your county clerk's office.

That way you will never be sued personally either.

See the chapter on Taxes for more information on this.

JIM & GLORIA

Jim and his wife Gloria lived in Houston. They had a nice one-story home where they cared for each other, as they were both in early stages of dementia. Family that lived nearby would check on them whenever they could, and a neighbor, who was a very good friend, came over every day around lunch time to check on them. The neighbor would call one of their sons with status reports whenever she had concerns.

One day Jim drove home from the grocery store, leaving Gloria at the store, without realizing what he had done. Somehow the neighbor found out that she was stranded at the store, and brought her home. The neighbor also discovered that they might have been taking the wrong prescription medicine, or not taking any at all. BIG RED FLAG! One of the daughters belonged to the same church as us and asked Marilyn for advice. After a few weeks, it was clear to the daughter that Mom and Dad both needed a place where they could get the help they needed.

We had one large bedroom with a private bath that was vacant. One day they arranged for Marilyn and I along with all the family, to meet at Jim and Gloria's home in Houston. The family showed up with a truck, and we packed them up and brought them to our place in San Antonio, caravan style. Gloria was confused, but Jim was downright displeased with the whole situation, and we had to stop several times on the way from Houston to settle him down. He and Gloria were riding with one of the sons.

It took a week or so for Jim to settle down to where he wasn't angry anymore, but still confused, and wondered where his car was. But, after a couple weeks his medications were doing their job, and we were doing ours. He liked to keep busy, and helped around the house. He took the vacuum cleaner apart a few times, and TRIED to put it back together. He also helped with the dishes. He wanted to help out in the yard, but would wander a bit if we weren't paying strict attention to him. So, we built a privacy fence, completely enclosing, and securing our large back yard.

Jim could then spend as much time as he wanted on the large, comfortable deck, and in the yard. Most of the time, Jim was just getting away from Gloria during the day, as her dementia was progressing more rapidly than his. He would sit for hours in the shade on the deck, drinking iced tea, and just enjoying the peace and quiet. Gloria would stay in the house, watching TV or reading, but she was always asking where Jim was. If he came into the house, she would tell him to get her something, or nag at him about something else constantly. But she was pleasant and polite with everyone else in the house.

When we went to church, Jim and Gloria would sit with us instead of their daughters' family. Their daughter and son-in-law would come to our house and visit a few times per month.

Several (maybe 6 or 7) months past, when one evening Gloria was nagging Jim after they went to bed. Jim gave Gloria a push with his foot and she fell off the bed, breaking her ankle. One of our caregivers got in there when she heard the commotion, and woke us up right away. We got Gloria to the emergency room. They put pins in her ankle, and released her back to us a couple days later.

We had a long talk with the family and showed them the video from the security camera in Jim and Gloria's room. We had another large home we had acquired about a half mile away from ours where we had three caregivers, two residents, and one extra room. Gloria moved in over there.

Jim stayed with us. Gloria got the rehab care she needed. Jim got the peace and quiet that he needed.

However, the daughter did not have any peace with the situation. She decided to take control. Her kids were off to college or out of the house most of the time, so she moved Mom and Dad in with her and her husband. That was fine with us, except she talked two of our caregivers into going with them. They soon bought a second house, and moved Mom and Dad and the caregivers into that house.

Marilyn was able to replace the caregivers rather easily, and we got two more residents within a month.

CHAPTER SEVEN

REGISTER YOUR BUSINESS NAME

Make sure you register your business name with your state's Secretary of State, or other governing authority.

This would require that you do some research for your business name. Check a number of things; your name availability in your state, website domain name, something easily recognizable, suitable, appropriate, and catchy if you can.

Most of these things can be done online, sometimes with a small fee to your state for the name availability. The registration fees vary from state to state, and will require some legal paperwork. You might be able to do it yourself if you feel comfortable doing it. If not, a good business attorney can assist you.

I also recommend that legal documents for establishing your business be recorded at your county clerk's office, in case of any hassles down the road. For example; sole proprietorships do not have to be registered, but someone else may already be doing business under that name. There will be another fee for recording the documents.

After you have selected and registered your business name, open up a separate bank account under that name so that your business income and all of your business expenses are separated from your personal finances. You will need to get a Federal Tax Identification Number from the IRS in order to open the account. Also, fairly easy to do. You and your tax preparer will be very happy!

SHALEY

Shaley was one of the three Silver Dancers that Monica had connected us with. It had occurred to us that if all of our caregivers were Silver Dancers, and we had season tickets to the Spurs, that on game nights there would be no caregivers at home. So, Marilyn and I decided that once the NBA season started, we could only keep one of the girls.

After a few weeks of having all three girls in the house, Ashley and Allison indicated that they each had somewhere else they could go. Shaley had bonded with Marilyn, and the residents, and really wanted to stay.

She had been adopted at an early age, and raised by a very nice couple who lived in Kansas City. She had a fiancé who lived and worked in Kansas City as well. But, her desire to be a dancer brought her to San Antonio, and then to us.

We brought in a couple more live-in caregivers, so that no one had to work more than 2 or 3 days per week. Shaley also worked evenings as a hostess in one of the nicer restaurants near us, to make extra money.

Her relationship with the ladies was special. She really enjoyed being with them and interacting with them, even on days when she was not working. She wasn't excited about the cleaning chores, but cooking was fine, and of course the ladies loved her.

At the end of the NBA season she decided to move back to Kansas City. She did, however, have to come back to San Antonio a few months later. During that trip, she called Marilyn, and asked if she could come out and take the ladies on a picnic. Marilyn said, "Of course you can!" She spent the afternoon with the ladies, and some time with Marilyn and I before she left.

An interesting sidebar about this story was that Ashley called about a year later. She asked if she and a young man she was dating could meet with Marilyn and I. We said yes, and spent a couple of hours talking to them. Ashley confided in Marilyn that she wasn't sure if this was the right guy for her, and wanted Marilyn's opinion. I don't know what happened afterward, but we felt honored that after only a few weeks of being in our home, Ashley sought our approval and counsel, on such a personal matter.

We came to realize that our ministry in this venture isn't only to the residents and their families, but to the caregivers as well.

GOLDEN EGG!!!!

CHAPTER EIGHT

COMPENSATION

In order to determine what our bottom line was going to be, we needed to do some math. As any for-profit business model would do, we had to figure out our margins. How much was it going to cost us to run this business.

It was our private home so we already paid for the mortgage and casualty insurance. We also paid for utilities; gas, electricity, sewer and water. Maintenance, such as lawn care, A/C and heating service, pest control, appliances, and normal wear and tear on the house were coming out of our pocket already.

However, we know that as people get older, their physical requirements change. Instead of keeping our heat set at 70 degrees and A/C set at 76 degrees for energy saving purposes, we would need to keep the areas where our residents live, a little warmer in order for them to feel comfortable. That means a little decrease in cost as far as A/C goes, but a lot more cost for the heating.

We would also need some additional insurance for the business. Our appliances and our house in general would get more wear and tear. We would use a lot more water, so our sewer bill would increase accordingly. There would be more lighting and TV playing, so our electricity use would increase. So, we estimated that those costs would go up around 30 to 40%.

After putting a 40% increase into our budget for those items, we had to estimate any additional costs we would have.

In order to figure out the cost for food, we needed to do a few things. Number one was to work out dietary changes. Figuring out a nutritious daily, weekly and monthly menu for our residents took a while, but we came up with one that fit the bill for a basic needs resident. Any special dietary needs for an individual resident would have to be paid for by the resident's family.

So, now we had established that there would be a base level charge for residents with basic assistance needs. And, as level of care for the residents increased, we would have to raise our monthly rates for those residents. If it was going to cost us more money, that was a no brainer. If it would mean more work for us as a caregiver, we would have to figure out ourselves what that would be worth.

After doing all the math, we estimated that fixed expenses would run us about $800 per month more than what were currently spending per month no matter how many residents we had. The cost for food per resident would run us about $300 per month, including a few meals per month; going out to a restaurant after church, or while shopping, for special occasions, or just for fun.

Laundry and cleaning supplies, including wipes, gloves, etc., would probably cost us another $100 per month.

And, the up-front costs of ADA compliance to the house, equipment; such as hospital beds, mattress covers, security monitoring and other miscellaneous things all needed to be figured in as well.

We set our base level care rate at $3,000 per month. We also came up with a list of other needs which would require level increases of $500 per month for each additional level of care.

That was based on our local and regional average for eldercare that other facilities charged, and that the fact that we wanted to be slightly lower. Making sure our home would be a more attractive choice for private pay residents.

If we did all the work ourselves, 24/7/365, and only had one resident to care for our bottom line for a basic level resident would give us $1,600 per month not including the up-front costs, which would vary depending on your house, amortized over the life of the improvement, or equipment.

That is the obvious business model.

Now, for a **"Golden Egg"**.

How big your **Golden Egg** is, depends on how many residents you can or want to care for, and how much help you might need or want.

The emotional and spiritual **Golden Egg** is the bond between you and the resident. Beyond the fact that you are now caring for someone who really needs your help, you are building a relationship with that person. They live with you 24/7/365 in most cases. They may, or may not know in their mind that they have a family, but in their heart, you become family to them.

The Residential Eldercare Home business is a huge financial **Golden Egg**. Your home has now become a place of business. All of the areas used for that business, and all of the expenses for that portion of your home are tax deductible, depending on the Business Entity you choose, for your Residential Eldercare Home.

You may want to consult with an accountant or tax advisor on the best way to handle these matters.

But, if 70% of your home is used for business, even if you use it as well, 70% of your mortgage, insurance, utilities, and maintenance are now covered by your business. In addition, you will now be able to deduct depreciation on 70% of your home as well. All of these deductions are right off the top of your income from this business.

You might consider as one option to rent 70% of your home directly to your business. However, that means that the rent may now be personal income to you.

If you decide you want help, you can do what we do. Give a live-in caregiver FREE board and room for 2 days and 2 night's worth of work. That includes light housekeeping duties as well. You can negotiate extra pay for extra days, and extra pay for extra residents or any combination that you want. You could also get a second or third live-in caregiver if you have room in your home.

We talked to the State of Texas Workforce Division and told them what we do. We then asked them what compensation to a caregiver who lives with us 24/7 and was free to eat 3 good meals a day plus a couple of snacks, which is what our residents get. They determined that alone would be worth around $1,200 per month.

The real work done by the caregiver usually amounts to about 6 hours per day of actual work. It's not hard work but it is busy work. Caregivers can sleep at night, they can read or do other things during the day, but they need to be aware and available to the residents on the days and nights when they are responsible for the residents.

DAD

My Dad was a very special resident. After my mother passed away many years ago, my two brothers lived with my Dad in his apartment in Wisconsin. It was a little crowded, but they made it work, since Jim had his own room in the apartment and Robin only slept there occasionally on the couch; as he had a room in the shop where he and Jim created and sold their sculptures. My brothers are both very talented chain saw artists, carving figures out of logs.

At first Dad was quite independent. He could still drive a car, and his mind was clear enough to get into everybody's business. My two sisters helped quite a bit also, but they both lived quite a distance away.

As time went by, Dad's cognitive memory and skills started to fade. He could no longer safely operate a vehicle, and did not like it at all when the kids took away his car keys. Under the care of a VA doctor, he was diagnosed with a few things that required prescription medication to calm him down a bit. These meds created side effects that required more meds. The spiral began and soon he was taking almost 20 pills per day, including a couple of narcotics.

My brothers and sisters couldn't care for him anymore. They tried a nursing home first. Dad's attitude got him thrown out. They then got him into an assisted living facility after getting more meds. He managed to stay there for a couple of years. His memory worsened and he became a fall risk, using a cane or a walker most of the time.

Marilyn and I visited as often as we could, Dad being in Wisconsin and us living in Texas. On our last visit, we could barely recognize Dad. He just sat in a chair all day by the entrance door.

I called my brothers and sisters and talked them into letting me take him to stay with us in Texas. I drove up to Wisconsin, told him we were going on vacation, put his things in the trunk of the car and brought him back with me. He was confused and anxious, and I had to figure out his meds on the way down to Texas.

We converted my office back into a bedroom for Dad, as the rest of the house was filled with residents and caregivers. Dad slowly settled in, but was still difficult. I found a new VA doctor here in San Antonio that worked with me for 6 months, getting him off all the narcotic prescription meds he was on. Then getting him off the meds for the side effects, down to 8 pills per day. His mind got clearer and he could walk without assistance again.

Dad accompanied me pretty much everywhere I went over the next 3 years. We became very close. Closer than I had ever been with him. If we were out and about and happened to go by a McDonalds or a DQ, Dad always wanted to stop and get an ice cream cone. He loved soft serve ice cream. When I was a youngster, Dad would ask all of us kids if we wanted to go for a ride around the lake on Sundays. We always wanted to go, because on the way back toward home, we had to pass the Dairy Queen. If it was a hot day, Dad would take the first lick off everyones' cone, claiming it was starting to melt.

He always worried about the boys. My brothers lived a pretty simple life. They lived day by day, working at the shop, fishing and hunting. They made enough money to get by, but Dad would kick in a few bucks once in a while to help them along. Especially for my brother Jim, who suffered from severe PTSD after he got out of the Army in 1972. That didn't change once Dad got down here to Texas. Dad couldn't help out financially, but if worrying was any help, Dad gave them all that he could.

If anyone reading this knows about ice fishing, you will get a kick out of this anecdote. One day while I was on the back patio of the house hand watering the plants, Dad was taking a little nap in one of the chairs with his face to the sun. I wasn't paying a lot of attention to Dad while I was watering. As I moved across the patio, dragging the hose behind me, the hose brushed up against the chair, jerking it slightly. Dad jumped up with a start, and raised his right arm quickly upward. I asked if he was all right and he replied "I thought I had a bite!"

Dad, all of his life, wanted to live on a farm again. I was born on a farm where Mom and Dad raised dairy cows, pigs, and chickens in Minnesota for the first 4 years of my life. He talked often about a small beef ranch he wanted to buy, before Mom put her foot down and moved us back into town, closer to her family.

After Dad had been here for a couple of years, I followed up on a promise that I had made to him. Marilyn and I bought a small farm about 50 miles north of San Antonio in the Texas Hill Country. It only had one house that was over 130 years old, and only had one bedroom. So, we moved in a 4 bedroom, 2 bath home and placed it directly west of our home under several huge live oak trees. We made it completely ADA compliant.

Both of our homes face north, overlooking a valley below and hills beyond. I built a big deck on the front of the house so Dad and any other residents could relax and enjoy the peace and quiet.

Dad would follow me around everywhere on the farm, supervising me while I put up fences, built sheds, chicken coops, a greenhouse, and turned the farm into our homestead.

After a little more than a year later, Dad passed away after a bout with pneumonia. Some of his ashes were spread here on the farm, and the rest are interned at Fort Snelling in Minnesota, as he had bravely volunteered and served in the United States Navy during World War II.

CHAPTER NINE

TIME

The amount of time you spend IN your business is up to you. The amount of time you spend ON your business is fairly minimal.

Short Term

It could take you a few months to prepare your home, and then secure your residents. You could be working on those items while taking care of the legal items on your list. The process of finding residents could be shortened substantially, if you are able to connect with referral agencies in your area.

Long Term

Your business plan, and your experience with the short-term aspects of this business will probably set the goal for the long term.

However, once you have acquired some residents, and some caregivers, you may find as we have, that we could do this for a very long time. I have often remarked, that when the time comes for me to need help, I can just move next door!

It's nice to have two or three **Golden Eggs** to put in the bank each month!

ANGIE

Angie was a very interesting woman who enjoyed serving and helping people. Whether it was her grandchildren, or elderly people with disabilities.

She was something over 70 years old, full of spunk and energy, and just dug right in no matter what the task was.

Marilyn first met her as a real estate contact. She ended up renting a home from one of Marilyn's investor clients. Her rental application showed that she worked for an assisted living facility, where she cared for 10 residents 24/7 with one CNA assistant.

When we opened up our second home in San Antonio (only a half mile from where we lived), Marilyn called her and asked if she would be interested in overseeing that home. There were a few things we talked about.

She lived about 20 miles away, didn't have a car, and needed to spend Sundays with her grandchildren. So logistically I needed to take her home, or to a bus stop early Sunday mornings before church, and pick her up later in the evening.

So, she would be in our Residential Eldercare Home 6 days and 7 nights per week. Basically, that was the same arrangement she already was doing at her current job. In addition to room and board, we paid her a salary each month, enough to cover her rent on her home, and a few other expenses she had.

She had a sizable pension coming from Hewlett Packard where she worked in management in California for many years. She sent that money on to her daughter who lived in California each month. We didn't know much about that job until a couple of years later, when she wanted to go see her daughter in California. Hewlett Packard arranged for a limo to pick her up, take her to the airport in San Antonio, fly her to California in their company jet, and a week later return her to us the same way. It turned out she oversaw manufacturing and technical start-ups internationally, and was fluent in six languages.

The first resident we placed in that home was my Dad. I realized that I could love him a lot more if he lived in a different home. He still came with me wherever I went, and I saw him every day. Angie took very good care of him.

When we got another resident, we found a couple more caregivers to help Angie with cleaning and other household chores. She still did all the cooking and took care of distributing medications. They also covered Sundays for us. However, all the residents still went to church with Marilyn and myself.

Eventually the lease ran out on Angie's home, but she still went on Sundays to spend time with her grandchildren, who she loved and spoiled constantly.

When we bought our farm, and said Dad would be coming out there with us, she agreed to come as well. We consolidated the residents and the caregivers to our original home in San Antonio until that house sold. Most of the resident's families thought that the additional 30 miles away was too far for their loved ones to be, and chose to find another place for them. That was completely fine with us, as we had anticipated that would be the case.

Angie did fine on the farm for a few months, but her daughter needed her in California. We wished her well, and thanked God for the time she was here.

CHAPTER TEN

BANKING

Your personal bank is probably fine for setting up your business accounts. You should have at least three accounts for your Residential Eldercare Home business.

The first account and primary account is the Checking Account. All income should come into this account either by direct deposit or by manually depositing the income yourself. All of your expenses should also come out of this account. If you choose to use accounting software like Quickbooks, these transactions may be easily downloaded from your bank, and manually or automatically categorized for tax purposes.

The second account should be an Escrow Account, where you monthly deposit enough money from your checking account to cover larger recurring expenses such as insurance payments or taxes, which may be quarterly or annually, and might create a cash flow problem when due. You can easily transfer funds from this account back into your checking account when it is necessary to pay these bills.

The third account may be an optional account where reserve amounts of resident's petty cash may be kept for larger personal expenses they might have. You can create sub accounts in your accounting software for each resident.

Certainly, small amounts of petty cash for toiletries, and outings can be kept by you safely in an envelope for each resident, with a record of their use and receipts.

You might, as we did, open a savings account as well to hold up to 6 months' expenses in reserve for some very rare lean times.

ED

Ed was one of our repeat respite residents. Respite care gives family members some time off, usually a week or two at a time. His wife had been taking care of him for many years. They were still a young couple in their 40's. Ed was a US Navy veteran. He was a deep-sea diver while serving his country. He suffered massive brain trauma while working underwater. A severe storm materialized rapidly forcing the ship to bring Ed up faster than he could decompress. The result was irreparable damage to Ed's brain and body.

Medically discharged with 100% disability, and under VA care, he and his wife built a custom home to fit his needs. The right side of his body was completely paralyzed. His speech was barely distinguishable, and at 6'-4" tall and a muscular 250 pounds, he was a handful.

But, with the strength he had on his left side, he could help with transfers from bed to wheelchair and back again. He was also on a catheter and had to wear Depends. After a few visits with us over a couple years, they decided to move back to Dallas, where other family members could help.

It was an honor to be able to help Ed and his wife when they needed it.

CHAPTER ELEVEN

INSURANCE

Since you are using your own home to conduct this business, you should check with your homeowner insurance for additional coverage on your policy.

Remember, accidents can happen. You want to make sure that you will be protected if or when something happens causing physical damage to your home and/or liability issues should be covered.

You may also need to check your auto policy for additional coverage, or raise the limits on your current policy, in case of an accident while any of your residents or caregivers are in the car with you.

You might consider an additional business policy, or an umbrella policy for higher levels of protection.

All of the additional costs for this protection are business expenses, which are fully deductible for tax purposes.

Another form of insurance is a security camera system in your home. If need be, you can go back and investigate what may have caused a fall or injury to a resident, caregiver, or guest in your home. We keep the receiver/recorder and a monitor in our office. We also have monitors, not cameras, in our caregivers' rooms, so they can keep an eye on things as well if they choose to do so.

In our case we have our primary residence on our small farm, and a separate home for our caregivers and residents. We had to treat our Eldercare Home as a rental unit, and insure it as such.

JOE

Joe came to us as a hospice resident. He had been released from the hospital under hospice orders, but he and his family did not want him to go to a sterile skilled nursing facility.

He had been living at home alone with his daughter who lived just a short distance away from him, and would come by every day to check on him. His mind was clear, but his body was failing. He loved to work on word puzzles, and could spend hours at a time, doing just that.

He was obese and diabetic. He needed insulin injections both morning and evening, and as required at meal times if his blood sugar tests were high. We did the testing and gave the injections, after his hospice nurse gave us training and instructions. We felt worse than he did when pricking his fingers for blood, and giving the injections in the stomach. He said he had become numb in those areas after so many years of having to do it himself. I still tried to find a different spot or finger each time.

He also required oxygen around the clock. He had a machine in his room at night that we would hook him up to. But, during the day he used a tank secured to his walker. We needed to monitor and chart his blood oxygen levels, and blood pressure morning, noon and night, which hospice provided.

Joe could toilet himself, but he needed help with showering.

Lastly, he was on several medications to treat whatever his other problems were. But his daughter would pick those up for him, and bring them over to us.

He was a pleasant man, and as I mentioned earlier, he liked to work word games, and word puzzles during the day. He didn't watch much TV, but he did go out on the front deck if the weather was nice and just relax.

When he was discharged from the hospital and placed into hospice care, the doctor had told his family that he probably had a few weeks or a couple of months at the most to live.

Under the doctor's approval, we recommended some changes to his diet, and some changes to his medications while he was with us. He lost some weight, regained some energy, and his spirit improved.

Joe stayed with us for nearly six months, and then returned to his home in better shape than he had been in a few years. His daughter resumed her daily visits to check on him.

That was another real **"GOLDEN EGG.**

CHAPTER TWELVE
CHOOSING THE LEVEL OF CARE

The level of care determines the level of what you need to charge the resident's family. If you check around for assisted living facility fees and find that the average monthly fee is $4,000 for a base level of care and you decide that $3,000 per month per person will meet your goals, then you may be able to fill your vacancy/vacancies faster. That level probably means the resident is completely ambulatory. He or she gets around on their own very well. He or she also needs no assistance with toileting, bathing, dressing, or eating.

Beyond that, the next level of care might require making sure the resident is using a walker or cane, as they have become a fall risk. They also might need help with bathing, dressing, or on a special diet. You might decide that you need an additional $500 per month to cover the extra care.

The next level of care might include incontinence requiring changing depends, cleaning and protecting skin from urine and fecal matter. Perhaps a wheelchair is necessary for mobility, requiring assistance to transfer the resident from bed to the chair and back again. Now we are talking $4,000 per month.

The level of care for hospice is much higher, but the hospice company will send CNAs and nurses, sometimes daily, to take care of bathing, changing bedding, and monitoring their patient's vital signs. They will also furnish, at no cost to you, gloves, pads, meds, lotions, creams, wipes, and any other equipment necessary for their patient.

We have had many hospice residents stay with us until they passed away. Many residents choose to live their last days with us as a family member might, rather than a sterile environment like a hospital or skilled nursing facility. One resident was with us a mere 3 days, another was here for 14 months.

It is completely up to you as the owner and manager what you are willing to do for the residents, making appointments with doctors, dentists, refilling prescriptions, driving and accompanying residents to their appointments. We charge an extra fee for those things. You might want to take them on outings including picnics, movies, shopping, theme parks, even plays or concerts. Just make sure that the person who placed the resident in your care, is comfortable with those activities.

Your residents will become attached and dependent on you, and your caregivers, as a child would be to a parent. Your residents will seem like family members.

PAUL

Paul was another resident that came to us for hospice. Again, he and his family did not want him to spend his last days in a sterile skilled nursing or hospice facility. When Paul came, he was barely responsive, heavily medicated, and bed bound.

Immediately, my wife Marilyn started to intercede for him. She held his hand and prayed with him for hours on end. Some of the time, he would respond with a nod, a sigh, or squeeze her hand. He spent less than 3 days with us until he peacefully passed away, still holding Marilyn's hand.

CHAPTER THIRTEEN

MARKETING

Website

Create a website for your business, with as much detail and as many photos needed to fully describe your business. Add hyperlinks to additional references or contact information about general information about Residential Eldercare Homes in your state. But, be careful not to redirect any visitors to YOUR site away from your website. Embed those references within your website. If you need help with creating your website, seek help from a professional, or ask one of your grandkids for help.

Your church

Certainly, your church family can provide a resource for residents. We put the word out in a church we had recently started attending, and the next resident we got was the Pastors' mother. She stayed with us for about a year before we asked that she leave. Her family understood.

There are tons of people that are looking for a home where faith is the foundation. No matter what denomination or religion you are, there is a need for these services. Our residents go to church with us every time we go. They enjoy getting out, and they enjoy the atmosphere. And of course, we go out for lunch afterward.

Your circle or network of friends

As with every business, some of your most loyal customers, and your first clients generally come from your closest friends, or your network. While you were still working for someone else, you might not have had the time or energy to care for someone you already know. They may be in an institutional setting, or an assisted living facility paying a huge monthly premium for their care. Chances are that they would receive better care, and be better off living with you for a lot less money out of pocket for the family.

Co-workers

Perhaps you or your spouse are still working. Spread the word around that you are providing a loving, caring and safe environment for elderly people to live in.

Maybe you are both retired or just want to change jobs. This could be the financial answer you need.

Senior Centers

Get to know the staff and volunteers at your neighborhood senior centers. Maybe you could bring goodies or lunch for all the guests, and explain what you are doing. Even if they aren't ready for your help yet, they might know someone who is. We did this and a wife who was caring for her husband for years, could no longer do the work. Not that it was so demanding, she was just nearly at that point herself.

You can also take your residents there occasionally as an outing for you and your residents. Your residents will spread the good word for you.

Referral Agencies

There are a lot of referral agencies that find places for loved ones. Once the elderly person needs more help than a home health professional can provide, or the person cannot afford to pay for the additional services, they and their families will start looking to referral agencies.

These agencies will generally send someone, maybe a team, out to your home for an evaluation interview. If they decide to take you on as a resource, they go through their files to find someone who fills the criteria for your home.

The agent will call you with a referral and set up a visit for the family. If after the interview, you work out a deal, the agency gets their fee. Sometimes it is flat fee, but usually it amounts to one month's fee that you receive. Since you will usually get 2 months in advance (first and last), you will already have the cash.

Relatives

They may or may not make the easiest or best residents, but they can still be a very good source for referrals. You may know many of their friends, but they have co-workers, acquaintances and church resources that you don't have. You shouldn't underestimate their influence and ability to help you in this endeavor.

Bulletin boards at your neighborhood convenience store or grocery store

Many businesses that cater to high volume walk-in customers have community bulletin boards that you could advertise or post a notice on. Some have FREE space, but many have a rental space where you can put a temporary or permanent flyer or a poster for a nominal charge.

Business Cards

You should always have a professional business card handy to give to someone when the opportunity arises. You can get them online or at Office Max or Office Depot in the printing center. Leave a few at the neighborhood Beauty Salon or Barber Shop. They can often be posted on one of those community bulletin boards I just talked about.

Veteran facilities – VFW, American Legion

With so many of our current veterans coming back from deployment with injuries both physically and mentally we tend to overlook our elderly veterans, who probably came home with the same problems, but were never diagnosed with any mental problems, because they didn't complain about them. They didn't complain because it was almost normal for them and their fellow veterans. They do however gather at their local veteran clubs and exchange stories while having something to eat or drink. It's a good place to network, but it is also a good place to share your appreciation for the sacrifices they made for their country. If you are old enough to remember; the World War I and World War II veterans came home as herocs, but most of us that served during the Vietnam Era weren't treated the same way when we returned home.

FRANK

Frank came to live with us 2 days after my father passed away. And since the only available room was Dad's room, I had to clear it out, and clean it, for Frank to move in. It didn't give me much time to carefully pack stuff up, and go through it. I went through some of Dad's stuff a few days later, and some a few weeks later, and the rest I haven't gone through yet, after more than 4 years.

Frank's daughter, Eva, was referred to us by one of the referral agencies. She called and talked to Marilyn at length, and brought her dad out the next day, along with all his belongings.

Frank was physically in very good shape. But his dementia had progressed to the point where Eva could no longer leave him alone, when she was working.

Frank was 71 years old. He was born in Guam, and had many brothers and sisters. Both of his parents worked to provide for the family, so his grandmother raised Frank and his siblings. The biggest problem with that was, she was blind. And Frank was a handful to keep track of, so she tied a rope around one of his legs, and the other end of the rope onto one of the legs on the table, when no one else was around to help her. He and his family lived on the island while the war going on all around them.

In 1959, Frank was old enough to join the Army, along with his best friend, and his brother. His brother eventually went to Viet Nam where he was killed in combat. His best friend got out of the Army after his first enlistment was over.

Frank, however got into the medical corps, and was originally assigned to the hospital in Pearl Harbor. The nurses far outnumbered the men there, so he stayed as long as he possibly could. Frank doesn't remember, but I think he married, and divorced wife number ONE there.

After getting promoted a couple of times, Frank was re-assigned to Germany. Again, he was assigned to the hospital for duty. This is where he met, married and divorced wife number TWO. However, Eva was conceived and born there in Germany.

He got promoted a couple more times, and re-assigned to a hospital somewhere in the United States. Neither he nor Eva remember where. But, he did manage to meet, marry and divorce, wife number THREE at that hospital. He does not remember anything about that marriage, or the fact that he has another daughter from that marriage.

He was promoted again, and re-assigned to Fort Sam Houston, in San Antonio, Texas. He worked as a radiology technician in the cardiology department at Brooke Army Medical Center until he retired as a Sergeant First Class, after 26 years of service. During that time, he met and married wife number FOUR.

Frank is not one to just sit around, even though he had retired. So, he got a government job, as a groundskeeper at the Fort Sam National Cemetery, where he worked for several years, and eventually retired. That eventually led to the divorce of wife number FOUR.

Number FOUR got the house, so he moved in with Eva. The divorce was finalized a few months after Frank moved in with us. He says he is looking for number FIVE, but Eva and us were not going to let that happen. So, we were very careful to alert the ladies at church, and our caregivers, not to give him any hugs or get too friendly.

So even after alimony, maintenance and child support, Frank was able to save a little money, and with his double pension, was able to support himself here, with no financial burden on his family.

Frank was with us for over 4 years, but Eva recently moved him to a facility closer to her, when it became apparent to her that his health was deteriorating more rapidly.

Frank, found it difficult to just sit around. He wanted to help anyone with anything, anytime. He helped with vacuuming in the house. He cleared the table and did the dishes after every meal. However, we needed to see that things were put away in the right places. He took out the trash, and kept the sink free of any dirty dishes.

Outside, Frank was a huge help. He got up at sunrise and hand watered everything in the greenhouse, and made sure the chickens had fresh water for the day. He usually hand watered the grapes in the small vineyard, and the fenced in covered area, where we raise blackberries and raspberries, daily as well. He used to hand water our orchard as well, but I have since dug in an underground, automatic watering system for all of our fruit trees, and the raised vegetable garden beds out there.

Frank also collected the fresh eggs, daily, and watered all the flower beds around our house whenever they needed it, and sometimes, even when they didn't need it. He also helped Marilyn trim the roses, and clean up the flower beds.

Frank was a joy to have around, and we took him with us quite often. He and Tom, who I haven't told you about yet, even went on a ten-day camping vacation with us. We each had our own tents, air mattresses, and sleeping bags.

I took Frank to all of his VA appointments (Frank and I now have the same VA Doctor), and refilled all of his prescriptions. I was also with him during his appointments to update the doctors on his behavior and physical condition.

Frank's dementia continues to progress, but at a slower rate under the current treatment plan.

Eva was very comfortable with our arrangement, but as Frank's condition worsened and she was finding it more difficult to make the trip out here to see him, she decided that a skilled nursing facility, just a few miles from her home, was more convenient for her. We have visited Frank in his new facility, where he is surrounded by nurses and a lot of people he doesn't know. He doesn't like it, and wanted to leave with us. We wish he was still here on the farm.

CHAPTER FOURTEEN

RESPITE

I haven't covered the respite care options yet. Respite can work both ways. Perhaps you have a resident that on occasion, you need a break from him or her. Perhaps the family can take their loved one home with them for a few days or a week if they can.

However, you lose money that way.

The most common way respite works, is that a family is taking care of the loved one themselves, but needs a vacation. You can offer them (if you have an available bed) services on a daily basis. The normal charge for that is 150% of your monthly (divided by 30) level of care charge. For example: You charge $3,000 per month for basic care, then the daily rate for respite would be $150 per day.

We have had many respite care residents. Some of them were one-time visits, but many were repeat respite residents. You may not have time to build a bonding relationship, but you will be surprised how attached you can get in just a few days. Each of them come with a story and a background that gives you enlightenment into their lives. They melt pretty quick as the level of care, and the emotion you share with them while caring for them, gives them peace and contentment.

There are a few cases however that backfired on us. Ones where the residents' level of care was not fully disclosed and/or the temperament of the resident was less than desirable. All of those were one-time respite residents.

We now try to visit potential new respite care residents in their own home before we make a commitment to provide care anymore.

The good news is that we have remained full capacity for several years now and haven't needed respite care income.

TOM

Tom is another resident who came to us through a referral agency. He moved in with us just a month after Frank had come to live with us.

He has three family members who are involved in his care; his ex-wife, Donna, his son Paul, and his daughter, Leigh Ann.

Tom is a native Texan, born and raised just an hour away from our place. He struggled with alcohol and some anger issues in his adult life. However, he was able to perform his duties and serve as a fire-fighter and a rescue diver in a successful career.

After many years of service in the Austin Fire Department, he was promoted to Captain, and commanded a station in the city of Austin. He received many commendations and awards for his courage and service during his career.

On Tom's last call, his station responded to a structure fire, with occupants inside. He and his men were able to get everyone out of the building, but Tom severely injured his back during the rescue. After treatment, the doctor ordered Tom to spend time in Rehab for his back pain. While in Rehab, taking a lot of meds, including pain killers, Tom suffered a mild stroke while walking around. Tom fell down and struck his head on the hard surface, resulting in severe trauma to the left front side of his brain.

After treatment for the brain trauma, he returned to Rehab, but was never able to return to duty. He was transferred to a nursing home at the young age of 55 years.

He had been medically discharged and retired from the Fire Department.

However, his family was disappointed with the treatment he was receiving at the nursing home. He was on a lot of pain medication, including several narcotics, and then other medications to combat the side effects of the narcotics. He spent his days sitting in a chair outside his room, barely able to communicate with, or even recognize his own family.

When Leigh Ann called Marilyn to ask if we would be able to care for her dad, Marilyn asked if she, her brother, and her mother, could bring Tom out for a visit. They all came out a few days later. We did our interview with them, out on the deck in front of the house, overlooking the valley below, and with dogs, cats, and chickens running around in the yard.

Tom could barely walk without his walker, or assistance. After talking for about an hour, Tom looked at his son, Paul, and said, "If I lived here, could I get my life back?" Everyone teared up. We moved him into our vacant room, next door to Frank right away, and Paul brought out Tom's personal belongings the next day.

After several months, working with Tom's new doctor, we were able to wean Tom off all of the narcotic pain killers, and most of the other meds. He now walks freely, without assistance around the farm, and wherever we take him. I take him to all of his appointments, and refill his meds. We all, recently attended his grandson's 1st birthday party. It was a large family gathering, and many of his family and friends were amazed at his improvement.

Tom continues to improve each day, carrying on conversations with caregivers, residents, and on the phone with Leigh Ann.

He and Frank were good buddies, and he is now very good buddies with one of our caregivers. They take several walks outside each day.

We look forward to years of having him on the farm with us.

CHAPTER FIFTEEN
LONG TERM / SHORT TERM

Is this a short-term solution to your overall plan or a long-term solution? How about for your residents? Are they there for a couple of weeks or many years? Are you providing respite services or hospice services?

These are very important questions you have to ask yourself and your family. Is this strictly a business opportunity for you, or is there more to it? For this business, the MORE has to be the definitive factor.

You may need this kind of facility someday yourself! I intend to just move next door when that happens to me. You might want to just stay at home!

Therefore, look at this as a long-term business adventure. The additional income is great; you can eat with the residents if you want to, and someone else may have prepared the meal, you have help with housework, and may even have help with the yard work as well.

Keep in mind, that if you have a large enough home, perhaps a married couple as caregivers might work out for you. Never hurts to have a handyman and a handy-woman around when you need them.

A FEW SHORT-TERM CAREGIVERS

I had been doing the majority of the caregiving during the first 18 months here on the farm. My dad, and the guys were pretty easy to care for, and I could take them with me whenever I had to go somewhere.

However, we were about to get a new resident who was going to need more care than the guys. So, Marilyn put an ad in Craigslist for help. She got many responses, and had several of them come out for interviews.

I was desperate for help, so Marilyn and I took that into consideration when doing the interviews.

After talking to their references and doing background checks, we tried a few on a 2-week trial basis. It was good to be able to sleep at home for a change, but that was about the extent of relief that I got.

We went through four candidates, giving me about 2 months of some help, before we finally found someone who made it past the 2-week trial period.

We now have 3 very responsible live-in caregivers, giving us, someone caring for our residents every day and every night, after building a tiny house for additional accommodations. And all of them appear to be long-term, since they all have part-time work on their days off for the income they need to not only meet their immediate needs, but allowing them to save for the future.

Consider YOUR needs carefully and the personalities of your residents, and use that criteria when interviewing caregivers.

CHAPTER SIXTEEN

RESIDENTS

There is a reason I have waited until now to talk about residents. You have read about some of the residents we have cared for in previous chapters. I wanted to give you a few examples of what we have experienced in our business. The elderly we care for come to us because they are suffering from Alzheimer's, Dementia, Brain Trauma, other Disabilities, or just plain tired of living alone.

Alzheimer's and Dementia are progressive and aggressive diseases that attack the brain and body organs and there is no cure, just medications and treatments that slow things down.

But all of our residents receive the same love and care that we would give our own family, no matter what their illness or how long they stay with us.

And if they pass away while under our care, we grieve for them as we would for any member of our family. But then we have room for someone else who needs our help.

You absolutely have the choice when it comes to residents. You can be very picky about who you want to share your home with. Some providers choose only men or only women. Some choose their residents by the level of care they need. Others go by the short term or long-term care method. And still others just see a need and fill it.

We always recommend a two week evaluation period no matter what criteria we chose to use. Within that first two weeks you will be able to tell if the resident is the right choice for your home. If we feel the resident does not fit, then we calculate the period he or she stayed with us on the daily rate, and refund the balance of the up-front money we were paid to the family.

However, that doesn't work very well if we had to pay a referral agency for the referral. We wait to pay the agency until after the two-week evaluation period is over. If the referral agent was misleading the resident's condition or behavior, the agency will not be paid, and the agency will have to deal with the family again.

Most of the resident's stories I have shared so far have been positive. That has not always been the case. We have had to deal with angry and aggressive residents, who we let go immediately as soon as that behavior surfaced. In one incident, we had to call 911 and let the EMTs and the Shcriff work it out. We will not tolerate those behaviors in our home, as it could lead to safety issues for the resident themselves, our caregivers, our other residents, or our property.

Remember, it is your home and your business to run as you see fit. You set the boundaries and the guidelines for this business. Be up-front with the referring agencies and the family members who are placing their loved one in your care.

XAVIEN

Xavien answered Marilyn's ad for a live-in caregiver, as he was studying to be a minister, and was looking for a place to live for several months. He and his fiancé chose courtship and abstinence until they were married.

Xavien was another special case. He was a former point guard who played in the D League for the Houston Rockets. A 6'-2" guard who could dunk the ball and dribble 2 balls at the same time. However, the lifestyle of an NBA player was not conducive to what he felt God's plan for him was.

He and his fiancé were trying to save money, so he let her have his car while he stayed with us. She came out to visit a couple times a month while he was with us. Occasionally she would come out on Sunday morning and they would go to church together in Austin.

If he didn't go with her, he enjoyed going with all of us to our church, which was situated on a 70-acre ranch and retreat center with a huge dining hall, tennis courts, basketball court, swimming pool, soccer and football field. One of the ministries at the ranch was providing counseling and rehab for young men with addictions, with living quarters on the ranch. We all enjoyed interacting with the young men in the program. Some of them still stay in touch with Marilyn and myself, even after completing the 12-month program.

A few times per week, I would take him to our church where he would put on a clinic with the young men and boys who wanted to play basketball for a couple of hours in the evening. A few of the girls showed up to play once in a while also.

He was OK with the residents and very responsible, but we and he knew it was only temporary, and it did give us a break while he was here.

CHAPTER SEVENTEEN

FAMILY MEMBERS

Family members can be a blessing, or a curse.

Most of the time the families are very supportive and grateful for the environment and care that their loved one is getting.

Other times……………..not so much.

We have had to let go of residents when the problem is really with the family. In some cases, they wanted to micro-manage their loved one's care, even if it contradicted with our policies or the doctor's recommendations.

In a couple of cases the family would just show up with a bunch of relatives or friends and want to throw a party. In those cases, we didn't let the residents go, but we put strict boundaries on the family visits. And this goes for friends as well.

In most cases, the family members have been very easy and pleasant to work with. They soon see that their loved one is being cared for with love and respect. They also realize that their own lives have become less complicated and they have some newfound freedom.

You might also consider asking the family members to delay visiting their loved one for the first 2 or 3 weeks, allowing their loved one to adjust to their new environment and caregivers.

Remember again, this is your home and your business to do with and manage as you feel fit.

LILI

Lili came to us through a referral agency. Her daughter had a power of attorney to act as her representative. Lili was the surviving spouse of a US Navy veteran. She was 87 years old, but seemed to be a good fit for our home physically and mentally.

She did however want a nicer private suite with a private bath. We had one available that I was using for myself as we did not have another caregiver in that home.

We had only myself and two gentlemen in the house after my father had passed away. The guys were pretty easy to care for, so with Marilyn's help, I took care of them 24/7 for nearly 5 months here on the farm. My wife was right next door, so during the day she assisted me in caring for the guys.

I moved into the only other private room available, sharing the other bath with the guys.

Lili's family moved her in with all of her own bedroom furniture and her personal belongings. I could tell by her clothes that she might be a little higher maintenance. She had been a homemaker her entire marriage. She met and married her husband in Greece where she was born, while he was stationed there during World War II.

Lili had never been employed outside the home her entire life, but was well educated and raised 2 daughters and 3 sons. Her husband had opened up a few car dealerships after he got out of the Navy and was doing quite well financially so there was no need for her to work.

During the first interview when her daughter said that they were not able to pay the full amount until they got money from the VA, I had to ask what happened to all the money. She then confessed that one of the sons, who lived at home all his life, had some issues, and had stolen everything of value; cash, jewelry, furs, guns, and electronics. He had also drained her bank accounts to satisfy his habits.

The family was not aware of this until Lili's health started to fade, and she was needing help from her daughter to keep up the housework and some other duties. They needed to sell her house in order to continue paying for her care. The son went to live with his brother in Oklahoma for a short period, and is now in a care facility in Oklahoma as a result of his choices.

Talk about a family problem. We got drug deep into all of the dirt with Lili's family. Bless her heart though, Lili really didn't know anything about all the drama and problems. At first family members were coming every few days, then maybe once a week, then skip a couple of weeks, then just once in a while. Her daughter gave me a debit card to pay for doctor and prescription co-pays, and personal items for Lili.

I took Lili to all of her doctor appointments, called for and picked up her prescription meds from the pharmacy, and Marilyn and I took her and the guys out on a fairly regular basis to eat, and went to church together every Sunday.

Lili had a few emergency room encounters. A couple of times she was transported by EMS after a 911 call. Other times I took her myself when it was not life threatening.

She became incontinent and a little more recluse after about 12 months. She no longer wanted to go anywhere or even outside on the deck, where she used to spend hours every day reading or petting one of the cats here on the farm.

After about 16 months with us, a bout with pneumonia sent her to the hospital again. While in the hospital the doctor suspected that she may have suffered a slight stroke as she could no longer support her own weight to walk.

The doctor recommended hospice care for Lili upon discharge. She returned to us, but hospice took over her care. They came to our home on a daily basis, sometimes twice a day for the first few weeks. Then Lili's health gradually started getting better. She could still not walk, but could help us with transfers from bed to wheel chair and back again. Hospice then turned over some of the care to us, and they only came out 2 or 3 times per week, with a few phone calls to see if we needed anything.

Lili finally passed away in her sleep one night, after spending 14 months in our home under hospice care, and spent a total of 30 months with us.

Her daughter was in the US Virgin Islands, visiting Lili's grand-daughter, on vacation, when Lili passed away. But her daughter had left me an envelope at her place of business with instructions for me, if I needed them. I had picked them up a few days earlier, as I saw Lili deteriorating rapidly. I made all the calls around 3:00 AM and by 7:00 AM Lili had been taken away. The family came over and picked up the items they wanted, after they returned from their vacation.

They were very grateful for all the care and help we had provided.

The 2 live-in caregivers (Analiza and Isabelle) that were helping us care for Lili, and the guys, were both heart broken, as this was their first time where someone had passed away while they were here, and they had grown very fond of Lili. They re-focused on caring for the guys, and their own interests on their days off.

CHAPTER EIGHTEEN
CAREGIVERS

Many of our caregivers have come from ads we placed on craigslist offering free room and board 7 days a week, in exchange for 2 days and 2 nights' worth of caregiving and light housekeeping. That leaves them 5 days per week for other part-time employment, which meets their financial obligations.

The only financial cost to you is for the food they eat. And that is from the same menu and grocery list that the residents eat. Anything else the caregiver wants, he or she needs to buy for themselves. That usually means junk food and sodas, not to be eaten in front of or shared with the residents.

You must do a thorough interview, including background checks, and calling references. Your initial contact with them is usually on the phone. Do as much screening on the phone as you can, asking some tough questions as well. Why have them meet with you, wasting your time and theirs if the phone call can qualify or disqualify them first. Take notes on the phone call, so you can do follow up questions in person later. Sometimes the answers change! RED FLAG!

My wife takes the calls, and is very thorough. I usually do the face to face interview along with my wife, as I am the primary caregiver for our business.

During the face to face I sometimes jokingly say "Eldercare is a lot like childcare, only the diapers are bigger." I watch for the reaction. I don't want them calling me every time someone needs changing.

The most common thing we have seen is the caregivers' need for a place to live. They are usually coming off of a bad relationship and need to get away for a while. Sometimes they are just trying to save some money by working for their board and room which is worth about $1,200 per month here in Texas. It may be worth a lot more where you live.

If you feel good about them on the phone, invite them to come to your place for the face to face interview. Do they have any caregiving experience? Can they cook and clean? After you have talked to him or her and still feel good, introduce them to the residents and give them a tour. Still feel good, then let them know you will be calling their references, and doing the background check. For that you will need their full name, birth date, social security number, places they have lived in the past few years and contact information. Ask them about their social media activities, Facebook, Twitter, Snap Chat, etc. and then check them out, as most employers do now.

Remember, you are bringing them into YOUR HOME to live!

ANALIZA

Analiza was an energetic young US Navy veteran. She was recently divorced with an adult daughter who lived about 25 miles away. She needed a quiet place to live, but needed to stay busy at the same time. Being a caregiver at our home was a perfect fit for her at this time in her life.

Before she started for us, she committed to spend at least a year with us. That was great, as we were really needing some help, after a long period of doing all of the caregiving. Now, that was our choice, using the money we would have spent on a caregiver, to build up reserves, and pay down some debt.

We agreed to give her free board and room for 2 days and nights of caregiving, and then paying her cash as an independent contractor, for any additional days and nights that she worked. Since the house was now full, I slept on the couch on the nights that I worked. Which, Praise God, were only a couple nights per week.

So, Analiza was able to visit her friends and daughter a couple days a week, and enjoy a little freedom, having a few less worries in her life.

She was very responsible, but occasionally needed to respond to her daughters needs for care, as she was dealing with some issues of her own. Our schedule was pretty flexible, so we were able to switch days with her at those times.

After several months, we brought in another caregiver to help Analiza. We had finished building a small guest house on our farm, and offered that home to Analiza, while she was here.

So now I only worked on Sundays, as we always took everyone to church, and out to eat lunch afterward anyway. Fixing breakfast and dinner wasn't that hard, and I didn't have to pull the night shift.

Analiza got a part-time job for a couple days per week to meet her financial needs, and things went pretty smooth.

We, however, went through a couple more short-term caregivers, during the next few months.

Analiza needed a couple of weeks off, early on, to travel with her family to Ireland on vacation. After she had spent more than a year with us, we gave her a 2-week paid vacation, so she could make that trip to Ireland alone a year later. She had developed a long-distance relationship and she wanted to see if it was still working. It was, as she confided in us, when she returned. A few months later, soon after Lili passed away, she gave us notice that she was moving to Ireland, and taking a caregiver position there.

ISABELLE

Isabelle responded to an ad that Marilyn had placed in Craigslist, after we had tried a couple of other caregivers, to help us and Analiza. She had some experience with caregiving as a mother, and was looking for a position that would provide her with a relatively quiet environment, in which to write. She was a well-educated young author, who was just finishing writing a science fiction novel, that was already sold to a publisher.

She also did research and wrote articles for a number of periodicals and newspapers that she had built relationships with over the years.

She thoroughly completed all of her tasks, on the two days per week that she was scheduled to work. She was totally absorbed in completing her novel the rest of the time. She appreciated and enjoyed her life here with us, and rarely left the house.

When she did leave the house, she went with Marilyn or myself, just to do a little shopping for herself. Sometimes she tagged along with me and the guys when I did the grocery shopping for the house. She took care of the guys when we went, and freed me up to do the shopping. They usually had lunch during that time, as it took me an hour or more to fill one or two carts.

She finished a contract to write an article for a magazine that focused on the long-term effects that the Olympics have on the economy and social aspects of the host cities and countries. Since the 2016 Summer Olympics were held in Brazil, her native country, it was of special interest to her. Her fee for that article gave her enough money to find her own place in which to complete her current novel, and continue writing her next one, which she had already started.

SUZANNE

Suzanne was another caregiver that responded to a craigslist ad. She had experience as a caregiver for a couple of relatives. And she had a wide variety of employment experience, working in radio broadcasting, marketing, and she was a self-employed grant writer.

She did a great interview and was able to start working right away. We needed someone to help Isabelle after Analiza left for Ireland, so she moved into the tiny house, as Isabelle was still comfortable in the large suite in the home with the guys.

Suzanne really got along well with the guys, but her and Isabelle didn't get along with each other some of the time.

Most of the disagreements were about cleaning up after each other on their days to work. My wife and I had to arbitrate and intervene every once in a while.

After a few months, Suzanne moved out, only to return again after Isabelle left. She only stayed for a couple of months again. She had found employment which didn't work out with her schedule here and was a long commute anyway.

We wished her well and found another caregiver to take her place.

CHAPTER NINETEEN

MINISTRY OPPORTUNITIES

The opportunities for ministry in this business are boundless.

Let's start with the family members who make the initial contact with us.

Marilyn will take or make the call, listen attentively to the person on the phone for a short while, then end up in a counseling session over the phone as she empathizes, sympathizes, and then offers advice and counseling to that person.

Generally, the family member is at wits' end in dealing with the situation. They don't know what their options are or they are afraid to hear what those options are. They don't know if they can financially support their loved one outside of their own home.

They may have gotten our contact information from any number of sources, and not know anything about us at all. Like I said before, my wife does a very thorough phone interview with everyone.

Since we are a private pay home, the cost to the family is a great concern for them. Even if the loved one that needs help has assets, in the long term those assets might have to be liquidated, leaving less of an estate to their heirs.

Even after their loved one moves in to our home, there is opportunity to minister to the family members. Educating them on their loved one's actual behavior patterns that family members deem as inappropriate at times, or different, and letting them know that these are symptoms manifested by their illness and age.

The resident may need constant reassurance that they need not worry about living with you. They will also need to be redirected when insisting on going home.

Not only family members, but friends of the resident, who are concerned about the care and the health of their friend, might need some counseling or ministry as well.

When things get a little tougher, you may need to minister to yourself or each other, seeking wisdom, strength and guidance from above.

TAMI

Tami was another caregiver who had unique qualities and skills.

She was a licensed LVN, who was working part-time as a hospice intake nurse for a large hospice provider in our area.

She was recently divorced, and a mother of an adult son, who lived at home with his father.

Our tiny-home was now available for a 3 day a week caregiver, and that suited her other work schedule, so she moved right in. She intended to be with us long-term and was able to get her own TV and internet installed, as our wireless network was not powerful enough to reach that part of our property.

Everything went well in the beginning. She was very conscientious and responsible. She maintained her own space and the residents home extremely well and fulfilled her duties exceptionally.

However, as time went on, we observed that her nursing background started to sterilize our family oriented home, both figuratively and literally. She scrubbed everything with harsh cleaners and chemicals, causing the residents home to smell more like a hospital than a home. She also decided on her own that the menu we had been using for years needed to be changed on the days that she worked, as she had special dietary needs and determined that her dietary needs and desires would better suit the needs of our residents.

Ironically, she was diabetic, and severely overweight. On days when she worked, she would make meals from scratch that included things that she liked to eat, including salads, pasta, carbohydrates, and desserts. On the surface that would seem like a good thing. However, the portions that she served were huge, and she would bake a cake or a couple dozen cookies every day, which would be consumed entirely in very short order.

Our male residents at that time all needed to lose weight according to their doctors, and were slowly doing so, but still had to lose from 10 to 30 pounds to get to their goal. They started gaining weight again.

In addition, she would no longer allow Frank to help with any of the work in the house, or on the farm, as he was diagnosed years ago as having contracted Hepatitis C while serving in the Army medical corps. She would not even touch anything he touched without wearing gloves or other protection, making him feel like he was some sort of monster (his words).

When I confronted her on these issues, she got defensive, and stated that as a licensed medical professional, she needed to do what she had been trained and taught to do, or her license could be in jeopardy. I reminded her that we were not a licensed facility, that Frank was allowed to roam about the farm and continue do the chores that gave him a sense of purpose and responsibility in his life.

She insisted that she had to do things her way.

I suggested that she do things our way, or take her license somewhere else.

So, she did. As I own a pickup truck, I even helped her move in order to expedite things.

CHAPTER TWENTY
TAXES

There are a lot of things to consider when it comes to taxes.

What type of business entity did you choose? Did you choose more than one? How does the money side of the **"Golden Egg"** finally get to you? Were your entities properly created and filed? Do you have other businesses that can be a division of, or merged together into one? Will you need to file quarterly? Do you have a state income tax? Are there any other filing requirements for your business, such as information reports?

All good questions that need to be answered.

Perhaps I can help a little. It is a little complicated, but well worth the trouble.

I personally chose a single member LLC for my direct business entity. For these purposes, we will call it Pleasant Acres LLC.

A single member LLC does not have a federal tax return filing requirement. It simply passes all income or loss on to a single member, which is usually an individual, which the IRS says is generally the case. But, in my case, I didn't want that income going directly to me as earned income, subject to FICA and other personal taxes.

So, I created another business entity, a Limited Partnership. The Limited Partnership had three partners. The General Partner was another LLC that I formed. The other two partners were Limited Partners and they were Living Trusts that I created for my wife and myself.

Here are the reasons behind my thinking.

Pleasant Acres LLC receives all the income from the residential eldercare business and passes it through to ACME Business Limited Partnership without having to file any reports or returns to the IRS. However, in Texas, we have to file a state return, but the income never exceeds the no tax due limit of $1,000,000 in gross receipts. We also have to file an Information Report each year to the great State of Texas.

ACME Business Limited Partnership files a return with the IRS showing income passing through to the three partners.

ACME Texas LLC receives a K-1 partnership form for the 10% share of its' income. And each of the Living Trusts receive a K-1 partnership form for 45% of their respective incomes.

ACME Texas LLC has two partners. The two partners are each 50% partners and are the two Living Trusts.

In doing this, I have created three layers of liability protection, and have been able to pass on all profits or losses to our Living Trusts. Living Trusts do have a tax liability, if they retain any of the profits. But, if the Living Trusts disburse ALL of the profits to the beneficiaries, the beneficiaries claim that income on their personal form 1040 return. However, the income is PASSIVE income, and not earned income, and not subject to the 15% right off the top self-employment income tax. One of the money parts of the **"Golden Egg"**.

Talk to your tax preparer and/or your attorney about any and all of these matters.

RON

Ron came to us by way of a private referral. His sister is the person that bought Lili's home. She contacted Lili's daughter, when Ron was getting released from the VA Hospital in Houston.

Ron had served in the US Army as a computer operator, and upon completing his enlistment, he immediately got a job with NASA also as a computer operator.

As a young man, he and his two sisters were very close. They often vacationed together, and one winter decided to go skiing in Colorado. After they left the lodge and driving home the snow started falling heavily, and they felt they should put the chains on for better traction and control on the road. As Ron was putting the chains on, an oncoming car lost control and struck Ron, causing massive trauma to his brain. He woke up three months later in the hospital with no recollection of the accident.

After a lot of rehab, he was released and went home. His sisters kept checking on him on a regular basis, but finally had to place him in a group home. He went through several group homes over the years, then after several trips to the VA Hospital in Houston, his daughters decided to place him with us.

His brain trauma was almost exactly the same as the trauma that Tom has. So, we began caring for him the same way we did for Tom. We got him a new primary VA physician and have begun weaning him off of some of his meds, and with help from his sisters, are getting him back on the recovery mode.

He has taken a liking to us, our caregivers, and to Tom. He also spends time outside on the deck, enjoying the fresh air, the scenery and the critters that inhabit our place.

CHAPTER TWENT-ONE

WHEN YOU ARE FULL TO CAPACITY

Celebrate!

Congratulations! What an accomplishment! You have achieved what few others will be able to do. That is, share your home with someone who really needs your help, and generate additional income to help you in your underemployment, and/or your retirement.

Waiting List

When you reach capacity for residents you can always maintain a waiting list. You will have attrition due to family changes or level of care changes. Keep good records on your leads, as they might not come with a referral fee to an agency.

Referrals

If you have inquiries from families for residents which do not fit your profile or your waiting list is full, you may be able to refer them to another Residential Eldercare Home in the area for a referral fee. That is another **"Golden Egg"**.

MICKEY, DAVID, ELLIOT, JOHN, JOHN & PAT

These five guys are our latest caregivers. Since we are down to just two mail residents (Tom and Ron) we have chosen to use just male caregivers.

Mickey was here while Tami was still here, and he was the caregiver living in the residents' home and covering all the night shifts. He is a retired electrical engineer and recently divorced. He has since, bought a small acreage lot a few miles away, and built a tiny home and has moved on with his life.

David answered our ad to fill Tami's spot. However, Mickey decided to fill that spot, and David became the live-in caregiver taking all of the night shifts. David was separated from his wife for a couple of years, with nine children, and thirty-six grandchildren. He had one son and family with whom he had been living with about forty miles away. He needed a break, and stayed with us for several months before moving back with his son.

Elliot took Mickey's spot in the tiny house, working three days per week, but no nights. He had a part-time job afternoons and evenings, on his other days, and was an excellent caregiver. We had no doubt he would be a long-term caregiver. Unfortunately, a customer at his other job recognized his work ethic, and offered him a better paying job assisting him in his construction business, and also had a place for him to live rent free. He gave us a two-week notice after helping us for about 4 months.

John (DJ) answered the ad for David's spot, and moved in right away. He is retired and divorced, in excellent health, and still works online as a computer consultant, and an online DJ, hence the nickname. He is also very conscientious, responsible, and an excellent caregiver. He has completely moved in and given us all the tools and household items that he says he will never need again, since he loves it here and will not ever be leaving.

John (Trucker) answered the same ad as DJ, and was pleased to find out that we still had a vacant room. After interviewing him, we decided that we would rather have all 7 days and nights covered with caregivers, and only have two residents to care for. Now my wife and I have only management responsibilities in the Eldercare Home here on the farm. Trucker is an online dispatcher for his families trucking business, and has been for years. This place suits his life style, and he has also completely moved in.

Pat is a retired military man at the young age of 60. He served 10 years active duty in the US Army. He then continued in the same job as a civilian for 11 years while serving in the US Air Force Reserves. He has taken over Elliot's role. He recently moved to Texas from Ohio, and was working in customer service at the Austin airport. I reminded him it would be quite a long commute. After touring our place, he said if he could live and help out here, he would quit that job!

CHAPTER TWENTY-TWO

EXIT PLAN

If you want to move to another home, you can do so without much difficulty. However, the family members of your residents will want to approve before you can transfer their loved one.

If you want to quit doing eldercare in your home, or scale back the number of residents, the answer is, simply ask the residents' family to find another home for them. You may be able to find them another home in advance and get a placement referral from that facility. Or as rooms become available, simply choose to not fill them.

If you do choose to quit, and downsize, try to sell your business, with your home. If you have good caregivers willing to assist you in that transition, it will add to the value of the business. You might be able to get a fraction of the gross revenues for a few years. Everything is negotiable!

PETS

Pets can be wonderful therapy animals. However, not everyone in the house might enjoy having them in the house.

Allergies, fear, or any one of dozens of reasons can be a problem for the rest of the residents or caregivers in your home.

Be mindful of how everyone feels about Fluffy or Fido.

CHAPTER TWENTY-THREE
REFERENCES

The following information was gathered by calling directly, and talking to the licensing authority for each state, as to requirements for an unlicensed residential eldercare home, as of the writing of this book in 2016:

Please follow up for any changes in regulations for your state.

These states require a license for every home:

California, Connecticut, Florida, Hawaii, Michigan, Minnesota, New Jersey, North Carolina, North Dakota, Oklahoma, Oregon, Rhode Island

These states will allow only one unrelated person without a license:

Kentucky

These states will allow up to two unrelated persons without a license:

Alabama, Arizona, Colorado, Illinois, Iowa, Missouri, New Hampshire, Ohio, Vermont, Wisconsin

These states will allow up to three unrelated persons without a license:

Arkansas, Mississippi, Nebraska, Texas

This state allows up to five unrelated persons without a license:

New York

The rest of the states did not respond to my inquiries.

SUMMARY

As I stated at the beginning of this book, discuss this business opportunity with your friends and family. Pray about it, and do what God leads you to do.

The rewards are significant, and could change a lot of lives, including your own.

We are now down to 2 male residents (Tom and Ron), and 3 very responsible male caregivers (Elliot, John (DJ), and John (Trucker) who cover all 7 days and all 7 nights.

My oversight and management responsibilities haven't changed, but the day to day operations now fall on my caregivers, allowing my wife and I the freedom to spend time together doing whatever we want to do. Including just staying home and enjoying the lifestyle we have chosen.

That is the real "GOLDEN EGG".

About the Author

Rick Lundberg is a Minister, a Veteran, a Husband, a Father, a Grandfather, a Great Grandfather, a Brother, an Uncle, a Godfather, a Caregiver, a Real Estate Broker, a Management Consultant, a Small Business Owner, and is now a Published Author.

Rick has had an entrepreneurial spirit all of his life. He was born in 1947 and raised in Minnesota. Then after 50 years of shoveling snow in the winter, he and his second wife Marilyn went on vacation to Texas in January of 1998, got to San Antonio and decided to stay.

Rick served a couple of years in the US Army as an Infantry Sergeant, and then as a SP5 Company Clerk in the 1st Infantry Division, stationed at Fort Riley, Kansas.

Then after earning a degree in construction technology, he spent nearly 20 years in architecture and structural engineering as a project manager, first as an employee, then self-employed as an independent contractor.

While still living in Minnesota, Rick started up and managed: an engraving business which evolved into a retail store in a strip mall; a property management and maintenance business which grew to 44 crews working in 14 states in the Midwest; a residential lawn service with around 50 customers; a small business management corporation; and a delivery company which served Sam's Club customers who bought in bulk.

After moving to San Antonio, Texas, Rick with help and support from his wife Marilyn started up and managed: an online real estate brokerage, listing domestic and international properties for sale. He proceeded to get his Texas real estate license and started flipping houses that he and Marilyn remodeled. After Marilyn got her Texas real estate license, Rick proceeded to get his Texas real estate broker license, and also got licensed in Minnesota and California to serve his investor clients. He, along with a few partners, opened up 2 real estate offices in San Antonio, which, when combined had over 100 agents; and finally started up 2 Residential Eldercare Homes. He currently manages 19 small businesses in Texas, Minnesota and Nevada.

Even though Rick and Marilyn have reached retirement age, and both being in excellent health, they continue to work in their businesses, including the Residential Eldercare Home, which they operate in a separate home, on their small farm in the Texas Hill Country, north of San Antonio.

The life that Marilyn and I are leading now couldn't get much better. God Bless!

www.ingramcontent.com/pod-product-compliance
Lightning Source LLC
Chambersburg PA
CBHW070249230526
45470CB00002B/541